KU-014-706

Contents

Social Science Library
Oxford University Library Services
Manor Road
Oxford OX1 3UQ

WITHDRAWN

RA
485
REB

Rebuilding Trust in Healthcare

Edited by

Jamie Harrison

General Practitioner, Durham
Associate Director of Postgraduate GP Education
University of Newcastle

Rob Innes

Vicar of Belmont
Part-time Lecturer in Theology
University of Durham

and

Tim van Zwanenberg

Professor of Postgraduate General Practice
University of Newcastle

Foreword by

Julia Neuberger

Chief Executive
King's Fund

Radcliffe Medical Press

Radcliffe Medical Press Ltd
18 Marcham Road
Abingdon
Oxon OX14 1AA
United Kingdom

www.radcliffe-oxford.com
The Radcliffe Medical Press electronic catalogue and online ordering facility.
Direct sales to anywhere in the world.

© 2003 Jamie Harrison, Rob Innes and Tim van Zwanenberg

All rights reserved. No part of this publication may be reproduced, stored in
a retrieval system or transmitted, in any form or by any means, electronic, mechanical, photocopying, recording or otherwise without the prior permission of the
copyright owner.

British Library Cataloguing in Publication Data

A catalogue record for this book is available from the British Library.

ISBN 1 85775 938 9

Typeset by Aarontype Ltd, Easton, Bristol
Printed and bound by TJ International Ltd, Padstow, Cornwall

Foreword

The context for this volume is clear – the Bristol paediatric cardiac surgery debacle, the Alder Hey scandal around retention and use of dead children's organs without consent, which turned out to be commonplace nationwide, and the Harold Shipman murders, largely of elderly women in their own homes, by their own GP. No surprise, then, that a first analysis suggests a breakdown of trust. But what the various authors argue for in this volume is both a more careful commentary and a series of complex responses.

First, 'trust' has not broken down, though it may be dented in many ways. Second, politicians have to carry some of the blame – and are, as a breed, far less trusted than doctors and nurses. Their own outcry, and their understandable response of adding more 'regulation', further 'targets', more 'accountability', has confused the public still more. The scandals, however awful, are simply not in the league of some of the terrible institutional abuses of adults with learning disabilities or with mental illness that were regularly tolerated by both politicians and healthcare professionals until the 1970s.

The retention and use of dead children's organs was appalling because of lack of communication and seeking of consent, no explanation, and individual and institutional arrogance – it was not necessarily always terrible in itself. The system failures (and individual failures) of Bristol paediatric cardiac surgery beg questions about clinicians who knew what was going on and did nothing about it, about a kind of professional arrogance, and about a lack of professional and managerial culture of co-operation and trust.

Of course, the Royal College of Surgeons, self-proclaimed bearer of standards, should have blown the whistle when it became clear what was going on, as should have the Supra Regional Services Advisory Group. But they did not. It was counter-cultural; each thought the other should not, and the Department of Health, which held the data, seems not to have recognised its significance.

So the change has to be cultural – one of leadership within medicine and management, and one of collective responsibility both for standards and for good working across teams and professional groups. More 'accountability' measures will only help to a limited extent. Politicians will be able to say they have 'done' something.

But real change is gradual, iterative, a response to a narrative, rather than to a single shock to the system. Many of the authors in this volume point to the importance of the story, the human tale. Many point out that we want to trust our healthcare professionals – and that many of us still do. But leadership and the new professionalism of doctors will need to be shaped by an ongoing telling of the story, from all perspectives, with the wider public. Patients to doctors; doctors to managers; carers to nurses; nurses to doctors; managers to doctors – in all these cases, different perspectives need to be brought to bear, and human leadership, with human frailty, needs to be acknowledged.

In the Jewish tradition, surgeons and physicians are held in the highest regard because they are thought to have been given the power to heal by God. In the Talmud we read: 'The school of Rabbi Ishmael taught: "And he shall cause him to be thoroughly healed ..." (Ex 22:19), are the words from which it can be derived that authority was given by God to the medical man to heal' (Berachot 60a). In Ecclesiasticus (Ben Sira 38:1–2) we read: 'Honour a physician according to thy need of him, with the honours due unto him. For verily the Lord hath created him.'

We need to trust our healthcare system and its professionals. For many of us, the values underpinning the NHS are the closest we come to shared values of civil society. If Rowan Williams, the new Archbishop of Canterbury, is to be believed when he argues that the nation state is giving way to the market state (Dimbleby Lecture, 2002), then that great post-war creation of an embodiment of shared values, the NHS, is under threat. The authors may well be right to say that 'professional and producer groups will have to supply a stronger and fuller rationale and ethos for the health service, and be able to articulate this in the public arena.'

Even more importantly, when they argue that 'Professional leadership may need to take up what government leadership finds it increasingly hard to deliver', they have hit on what is essentially the 'way through all this'. Professional leadership, cross-disciplinary working with patients and the public, is what will rebuild trust. Paternalism has to disappear. Blind trust is dead. This is earned trust, trust based on honesty, on listening, and on a strong sense of shared values. But it is possible, and desirable. And it is in the interests of all of us to work towards a new professionalism, with real openness, good communication, expressed and shared values – and a large dose of recognition of common humanity.

Rabbi Julia Neuberger
Chief Executive
King's Fund
May 2003

Preface

The theme of trust, or its absence, pervades much of modern-day culture. Onora O'Neill's timely *2002 Reith Lectures* caught the mood, opening up a discourse at a time when many are worried about the public's loss of trust in institutions. Equally, certain actions, especially from governments attempting to shore up trust, risk making matters worse as professionals find themselves overwhelmed by targets and micro-management.

In particular, the world of healthcare has suffered from a series of scandals involving individual doctors, teams and institutions. Highly publicised reports and court cases exposed the general public to accounts of medical activity that appeared shocking and which were, on occasions, criminal in nature. Certain sections of both the media and the political machinery made much of the failings of the medical profession.

The desire to write this book reflects a concern to continue a discussion on the nature of trust, how it operates in today's culture, and how it might be fashioned for tomorrow. We were concerned not to stigmatise any players in the system — whether healthcare professionals, patients, the Government or the media. We knew of cases in which doctors had been negligent and in which others had been tarred falsely with the same brush. We had met patients who had been damaged by their doctors. We talked to those who had tried to do their best and felt that they had been wrongly blamed when the system had failed. We came across criminals whose activity was an affront to society. We struggled over the question of whether our context was 'medicine' or the wider world of 'healthcare'. Although most of the high-profile events had involved doctors, there were cases involving nurses, and in both the Bristol case and the Alder Hey case, management contributed to the problem at the highest level. Equally, we wondered whether past governments had colluded with the professions by turning a blind eye to poor-quality practice, as part of a pact to contain costs. In the end, we opted for a title for the book that included the word 'healthcare', while at the same time conscious of the dilemma so posed, and of the complexity of the task set for our contributors.

It has been our increasing belief that trusting relationships are fundamental to maintaining and improving health and healthcare. It is our hope that trust, particularly between patients and their doctors, nurses and managers, can be rebuilt, even in this era of scepticism and suspicion.

Jamie Harrison
Rob Innes
Tim van Zwanenberg
May 2003

List of contributors

Richard Baker is Professor of Clinical Governance and Director of the Clinical Governance Research and Development Unit at the University of Leicester. He qualified in 1975 and worked full-time and then part-time in general practice until 2002. He has since concentrated solely on research into aspects of quality of care. His research interests include the meaning of personal care, methods of improving performance, and monitoring of outcomes.

Ruth Etchells was Vice-Chair of Durham Family Health Services Authority and Chair of its Medical Services Committee after retiring as the first woman and first lay Principal of St John's College with Cranmer Hall, University of Durham, which includes a training hall for ordinands. Her teaching and research interests are in literature, theology, and their interaction.

Jenny Firth-Cozens is a clinical and organisational psychologist and consultant to the London Deanery of Postgraduate Medical Education, after retiring as Professor of Clinical Psychology at Northumbria University. Her main interests are in team-work, occupational stress and patient safety, and particularly in the relationships between these areas. She was part of the expert group that produced *An Organisation With a Memory*, and is currently involved in research initiatives on reporting and learning from error.

Liz Haggard is a psychologist, and was chief executive of a community health trust for eight years. She runs workshops and conferences on local and national policy and service issues. Her special interests are new models of primary and community services, rehabilitation, expert patient approaches, outcome measures, personal effectiveness and the impact of the environment on patients, public and staff.

Jamie Harrison works as a general practitioner in Durham and as an Associate Director of Postgraduate General Practice Education in Newcastle. He has written on the careers of young doctors, medical vocation and professionalism. Together with Tim van Zwanenberg he received the Baxter Award from the European Health Management Association for their book *Clinical Governance in Primary Care*.

Louella Houldcroft trained as a scientist before turning to journalism. While studying for a degree in biology at the University of York, she took a year out to work at the Institutes of Oceanographic Sciences and Terrestrial Ecology. Formerly health correspondent with the *Newcastle Journal*, she is now the paper's investigative reporter.

Rob Innes was formerly a project manager with Andersen Consulting, and later became ordained. He is now vicar of a mixed housing estate parish in Durham and lectures in theology at Durham University. He has written on theology and psychology, personal identity, medical vocation and modernisation, and he co-edited *The New GP* with Jamie Harrison and Tim van Zwanenberg.

Di Jelley took a degree in sociology at Liverpool University and taught English in Mozambique before studying medicine at Nottingham University. She is a GP principal and also a lead research practitioner for North Tyneside Primary Care Trust. She works at Collingwood Surgery in North Shields, which since 2001 has successfully pioneered copying GP referral letters to patients as a routine activity.

James Jones is the Anglican Bishop of Liverpool.

Robin McKenzie is currently training for the ordained ministry within the Church of England, and is to be ordained in June 2003. His background is in business (engineering, sales and product marketing). His doctoral research interests were in business relationships between organisations, with particular emphasis on trust. His current research interest is in relating Christian theology and business.

John Newton is a Principal Lecturer in Sociology at Northumbria University. His main academic interests are in the organisation and management of medical professionals. He has recently completed a study of early retirement among general practitioners, and is currently investigating the development of research capacity in primary care.

John Spencer is Professor of Medical Education in Primary Health Care at the University of Newcastle upon Tyne. He is a general practitioner by trade, and has 20 years' experience in all areas of healthcare education, but mainly undergraduate medical students. His main educational interests are in teaching about professionalism (with a particular focus on communication) and community-based education.

George Taylor is Director of Postgraduate General Practice Education in Yorkshire and an Associate Dean at Leeds University. His academic interests centre on performance and clinical governance in general practice, developing teaching skills in primary care and the assessment of consultation skills.

Tim van Zwanenberg has had a wide range of experience not only as a general practitioner, but also as an academic and health services manager both in the UK and overseas. In 1996 he was appointed to the newly established Chair of Postgraduate General Practice in Newcastle, and from 1999 to 2002 he was chair of the UK Committee of General Practice Education Directors. He does his clinical work at Collingwood Surgery in North Shields.

Caron Walker is Research and Development Facilitator with North Tyneside Primary Care Trust – the first research primary care trust in the UK. Since graduating from Newcastle University with a degree in politics, she has pursued a varied career in the public and voluntary sector, and has considerable experience in the field of welfare rights. Completion of her MA led to a number of academic research posts focusing on disability, social care and health research.

Acknowledgements

We are grateful for the support and help of a wide variety of people in producing this book. In particular, we would like to thank the contributors for their enthusiasm and hard work. Many colleagues have helped to clarify our thinking by challenging us and asking questions. We have received helpful advice from Timothy Jenkins, Dean of Jesus College Cambridge, and from Madeleine Atkins, Pro-Vice-Chancellor of Newcastle University, who supervised Tim van Zwanenberg's doctoral thesis on doctors' revalidation. A group of clinicians, theologians, academics, patients' representatives and senior managers from the health service and the pharmaceutical industry participated in a discussion with us to answer the question 'Can I trust my doctor?'. They were Phil Adams, Richard Baker, Rupert Brereton, David Clough, Ruth Etchells, Josanne Hall, John Hamilton, Liz Haggard, Di Jelley, Robin McKenzie, Linda Redpath, John Spencer, George Taylor and Julie Toland. We thank them all for their thoughtful ideas and comments. We have, as ever, relied on our colleagues, patients and parishioners at Cheveley Park Medical Centre, Durham, St Mary Magdalene Church, Durham and Collingwood Surgery, North Shields. They have made us think, and have provided us with constant reminders of reality. We thank our wives for their support and for their patience in the face of dining-rooms submerged beneath papers. Gillian Nineham from Radcliffe Medical Press has encouraged us throughout. Angela McLaughlin has worked efficiently and with great calm and good humour to produce the final typescript, and our considerable thanks are due to her.

For our parents
Christine and Frank Innes
Aldyth van Zwanenberg

And in memory of
Herbert and Margaret Harrison
David van Zwanenberg

PART 1

Setting the scene

Trust is about people and relationships, and is experienced in the case of health-care by patients and their professional carers. The opening chapter is therefore written by a patient, and is followed by an exploration of how trust might be embodied and explained. The three subsequent accounts of recent high-profile cases of medical malpractice provide evidence of what happens when trust is misplaced. This group of chapters then ends with a description of how the system – the NHS and other institutions – has responded.

It is evident that patients perceive a weakening of the personal relationship that they have with their practitioners, and this goes for their friends and families as well. A sociological model of trust provides a template against which measures to restore that trusting relationship can be judged.

The cases of malpractice illuminate the complexities of that relationship, and provide some lessons on how trust is breached. Uncertainty about the systems that are meant to prevent and detect malpractice may be more appropriate than suspicion of the professionals themselves. Institutional factors can exacerbate the effects of an individual's malpractice, and medical culture needs to remain in step with public expectations.

The system has responded with a plethora of developments in the contractual, organisational and professional regulation of healthcare practitioners, yet there is doubt as to whether the techniques of performance management that are being deployed will have the desired effect.

The address given by Bishop James Jones at the memorial service for the Alder Hey children comes at the very beginning of this book – in order to challenge our presuppositions and make us think.

Honouring the memory: an address given by the Bishop of Liverpool at a service following the Royal Liverpool Children's Inquiry on Saturday 10 November 2001

Adrian Henri the Liverpool poet who died last year, wrote a poem called 'Christmas Blues'.

It begins as follows:

> Well, I woke up this morning, it was Christmas Day
> And the birds were singing the night away

> I saw my stocking lying on the chair
> Looked right to the bottom but you weren't there
> There was
> Apples
> Oranges
> Chocolates
> − But no you.

The poem ends as follows:

> So it's all the best for the year ahead
> As I staggered upstairs into bed
> Then I looked at the pillow by my side
> I tell you baby I almost cried
> There'll be
> Autumn
> Summer
> Spring
> ... And Winter
> − All of them without you.

It is the advent of Christmas that makes the heart ache for those who are no longer with us physically. Their spirit lives but we can no longer see and hold them. We grieve and feel bereft − bereft of their touch.

This is why the taking of our children's organs and tissues has been such an offence to parents and families. When your child is sick and helpless, you hold them to yourself to let them feel the warmth and reassurance of your body. When they die, the memory you cherish is the warmth of that embrace − body to body, flesh to flesh, heart to heart. The body − *their* body − weak and vulnerable, pressed against yours − strong and caring − hoping for a miracle.

When my own children were infants there was a moment when I came near to death after an operation. I remember holding my healthy children close to me in the hope that their health would somehow infuse my sickly body. How you the parents must have hoped that you could have transfused your own child with your own health and well-being.

So to discover that their body − so precious to your memory − has been violated leaves you understandably traumatised. Their body and the memory of their body are both marred. The discovery itself brings back their death so that the tragedy of yesteryear feels as if it happened just yesterday.

Of course, as you think back to those moments when you realised how ill they were, you remember how you longed for a miracle. The truth is that as you handed over your child to doctors and nurses, you did so with complete trust. At such a time we want the doctor to be God, to do the impossible, to deliver the miracle. Doctors do not take upon themselves a God-like status on their own − we confer it upon them for the sake of those we love and long to see healed. But when you discover what has been done without your knowledge, without your understanding, without your consent, you feel betrayed − so much so that it becomes difficult to trust anybody in authority. So here we are today doubly bereft − bereft of their touch and bereft of trust.

This lack of trust is the reason it has felt impossible to invite medical and management staff of Alder Hey to this service. I know that some parents are sad that they cannot be here — others could not consider it. I know that Alder Hey are sad not to be here. I know, too, that the Chair and the Chief Executive at Alder Hey are committed to the rebuilding of trust for the good of each individual and the well-being of the community that the hospital serves. This rebuilding is demanding and vital.

Alder Hey's absence is in itself a sign and a symbol that in our society those of us in authority who have power do sometimes forfeit the trust of those we serve. That has to be recognised. And it is recognised in this service.

It is not that the parents do not wish well the children and the staff at Alder Hey today. It is not that Alder Hey does not respect the feelings of the parents. Let this absence serve to remind all of us in authority of our duty to earn, to merit and to honour the trust that is put in us by those we serve.

This was very much the tenor of the Redfern Inquiry. Michael Redfern, who chaired the Inquiry, told me at the publishing of the report how deeply impressed he had been by the unfailing courtesy and dignity of the parents and by their courage and restraint in giving evidence. The report was a vindication of the parents from Liverpool and Manchester, from Wrexham and Preston, from Chester and throughout the North West. You knew that something was wrong and you would not take 'no' for an answer. Thank God for that famous Scouse stubbornness that challenges authority and champions the oppressed. Why? Because out of the depths of your experience, out of the dying of your children, out of the courage of your testimony, far-reaching decisions are now being planned that will change forever and for good the relationship between doctors and children and their parents.

We know honouring the memory of your children today in this place is both tearful and painful. But it is your tears that will wash away our fears for tomorrow's children. Your pain will be our common gain. Your children have not died in vain.

We thank God for each and every one, cherished today in this sacred place. We thank God that in him, in whom we live and move and have our being, we on earth are at one with those in heaven.

Our God knows the pain of finding the body of his own beloved child scarred and marred by human hands. He, the Risen One, is here to comfort us today.

> The hand with which he holds us bears the mark of cruel nails;
> the hand with which he leads us on holds us to the wounded side of
>   his body.
> He sees the tears in our eyes.
> Gently he wipes them.
> Our vision, blurred by weeping, begins to clear
> and we see again — the wonder, the miracle that in his other hand he
>   holds the one we love, the child we mourn, once lost and found, by
>   his side and safe for all eternity.
> Let the honouring of their memory and the remembering of their name
>   be a blessing to you,
> to us all,
> for all eternity.
> Amen.

CHAPTER 1

The patient's perspective

Ruth Etchells

> You can't trust the 'specials' like the old time 'coppers'
> When you can't find your way home.
>> (1919 song, *'Don't dilly dally on the way'*, by Charles Collins
>> and Fred W Leigh)

This chapter gives a patient's perspective on why trust between general practitioners and patients has been eroded. It portrays a weakening personal relationship between practitioners, their patients and the patients' families, and offers some practical guidelines on how this relationship might be restored to its proper strength.

I am that fortunate being, a satisfied patient – that is, over a period of years, suffering various blights and misfortunes and latterly a moderately serious chronic condition, I am conscious of having received excellent care from both my general practitioner and my consultant. So, robustly active, I write from no bitterness of soul.

However, during the 1990s, I was for some years Vice-Chairman of the Family Health Service Authority, which was responsible for all primary care in the Durham area. Even more to the purpose of this book, I was Chairman of the Medical Services Committee and therefore responsible for the handling of all formal complaints against Durham general practitioners. Therefore for quite a time I had both an overview of the doctor–patient relationship at the point where 'trust' was breaking down, and a public responsibility to identify the causes of this.

The complaints system is now quite different, and I am in any case no longer involved. However, my interest having been aroused, I have stayed in touch with the shifting patterns of the doctor–patient relationship. My perception is that it is very different now, and that the doubts and questioning – the 'non-trust' (a less virulent thing than *dis*-trust, but tending to the negative) which ten years ago shaped only a small percentage of doctor–patient relationships – is now significant in the context of a high proportion of them.

Cause and effect 1

The most common cause identified as the reason for formal complaint back in the 1990s, was 'poor communication' by the doctor – that is, communication about the diagnosis or course of treatment or his or her own intentions with regard to, or understanding of, the patient's state and needs. Certainly at the most practical and mundane level this failure was often apparent (and it still is). The patient's trust (or, just as frequently, that of the relatives concerned) was lost because the general practitioner did not explain in terms that were understandable, or if they were understandable, they were not 'heard', and he or she did not take steps to ensure that all comments were both understandable *and* heard. My own perception was that a major cause of this was cultural, the gap between the articulate world of the doctor and the inarticulate one of many patients being such that there was a huge linguistic barrier, and one that did not only involve the technical and non-technical use of words. So many patients from a less verbally assured culture 'got by' with their general practitioner as they did with so many authority figures in society – by maintaining a blankly unrevealing composure which hid their confusion, often near-panic, and lack of understanding.

In contrast, today at least as high a proportion of patients, at home on the Internet if they are not in the surgery, confront the general practitioner with almost the opposite problem, which is exacerbated in more privileged areas. For instance, Dr Furness of Greater Windsor commented that his patients 'frequently return home and use the Internet to check the ingredients in their prescriptions and compare waiting times.'[1] Such researches are by no means confined to the sunlit upper reaches of Southern English society – some doctors in the comparatively gloomy non-affluence of Peterlee in North-East England tell the same story. It suggests at best a use of intelligence by the patient to learn everything possible about his or her situation, but at worst it indicates a sense that they have not been told in the surgery all that they wanted and/or needed to know.

Other reasons for failure of communication in the past are well attested and frequently summarised. They include appalling pressure on the time and energy resources of the general practitioner, the speed of major developments in medical options, lack of adequate training of general practitioners in communication skills and (perhaps most of all) the burden of immense – often impossible – expectations of the practitioner among patients and their relatives. The Bishop of Liverpool summed it up clearly at the service following the Alder Hey Childrens' Inquiry:

> We want the doctor to be God, to do the impossible, to deliver the miracle. Doctors do not take upon themselves a God-like status on their own – we confer it upon them for the sake of those we love and long to see healed.[2]

Dehumanising the doctor

It is with this last aspect that I want to stay for a moment, because it is becoming clear that it was this impossible expectation, more than almost anything else, which was to move us towards the huge changes of the last ten years. From the patient's point of view, the combination on the one hand of a Welfare State medical system which meant that cost (*to the patient*) need never, it seemed, limit treatment, and on the other of advancing medical science trumpeted in the media as marvellously curing most previously intransigent disease, meant that the patient's expectation was such that in a real sense *the patient dehumanised the general practitioner.* That is, this was no ordinary human being with professional skills – this was someone whose *duty* was to work miracles, and who (by definition) had failed and 'broken trust', if the patient did not recover properly or, even more unthinkably, died.

'*Dehumanising the general practitioner*' meant assuming that he could be available 24 hours a day, that he could attend with equal immediacy and attention the patient with minor illness and the major emergency, that he could always diagnose promptly any problem, that he could always explain matters with the utmost clarity in layman's terms, and that he would never, never be impatient, rude or hurried.

Cause and effect 2

Given expectations which did not recognise the general practitioner as a human being with ordinary human limitations, it is not really surprising, to this patient at least, that general practitioners generally responded – *as human beings*. That is, they became exhausted by the imposition on their time and the burden of the 24-hour day, frustrated by the lack of public recognition of the limit of medical possibility, and angry about the sheer lack of human consideration on the part of many patients in their demands for attention to minor matters at unsocial hours.

And so what evolved was the changing pattern in general practice care that is now so familiar to us, and which began, at least, in defence of the 'humanness' of the practitioner. Twenty-four-hour care was modified so that night work became an emergency service not necessarily (or even probably not) involving the patient's own general practitioner. This allowed the doctor the joys of ordinary human life in off-duty hours – something we who were wilful patients had shown no concern about. However, its consequence has often been that the patient's 'own' general practitioner was not there at the most critical emergency moments – those life-saving (or, for the relative, death-facing) moments which bond together the general practitioner, the patient and the patient's relatives (who must never be left out of this equation) as almost nothing else can.

This severance of the connection between the general practitioner and some of the patient's most critical life moments has, of course, been compounded by the movement (not limited to large practices) towards suspending the personal doctor–patient relationship in favour of immediate attention from whichever partner happens to be on duty. I spoke in my first paragraph of 'my' general practitioner. I am one of the fortunate ones in that so far I have been consistently cared for, even in a large practice, by one particular general practitioner. Over the years we have learned to trust each other. Trust is a two-way quality and needs to be reciprocated if it is to be effective. Part of the general practitioner's task is to learn how far he or she can trust this patient. The move to a 'practice–patient relationship' rather than a doctor–patient one has resulted in a concomitant loss of personal engagement between doctor and patient – a loss of that personally developing *mutual* history that is essential to the establishment and maintenance of trust. And thus the fact must be faced that doctors are no longer fully trusted by patients who do not know them and who, equally, *they do not know and have not themselves learned to trust*. (A friend said to me, 'I always ask for – and get – the same hairdresser; I always ask for – and get – the same mechanic for my car, but in the most important area of all, my body, I can't be sure of asking for – and getting – the same general practitioner.')

Dehumanising the patient

At the same time, excited by technological advances, general practitioners began to regard their patients mechanistically (at least, this was the common cognitive illusion of many patients), seeing them as a series of challenging technological problems to be studied and resolved, rather than as living and feeling humanity with affections and sympathies, fears and anxieties which in fact materially affect the body's condition. Thus we find ourselves in the situation where the doctor, in response to feeling dehumanised, has in turn *dehumanised the patient*. Not to know the patients is to begin to dehumanise them — to think of them as the sum of technological issues is to complete the effect. This cyclical effect of dehumanising would, I think, have developed even without the additional pressure of a consumer-driven culture which applauds what the media call 'healthy scepticism' about the 'goods' on offer, a 'scepticism' which is more generally experienced as cynical — a self-righteous, judgemental culture which eagerly seeks to apportion blame. That is but the context, not the cause, and it simply heightens the attitude that now often exists between the medical profession and the patient. For a professional relationship that was based ultimately on *trust* has been replaced by a professional relationship that is based on *accountability*. The two are quite different, and the more emphasis that is put on the latter (as Baroness O'Neill pointed out in the 2002 Reith Lectures), the less 'trust' there is available.

Not Dr Shipman

The various scandals embroiling the medical profession in recent years — the Bristol Baby Inquiry, the Alder Hey Inquiry and, most dramatically, the Shipman Inquiry — have raised the profile of non-trust between patients, patients' relatives and the doctor. These affairs were to some extent extreme examples of what had become, as patients see it, a mind-set — a culture within the medical profession of obtuseness to human consequences. However, it is important to emphasise that the murdering Lancashire general practitioner is not the most common image for the patient even now. Patients do not enter surgeries expecting to be murdered (deliberately, at least). But — and this marks the huge change compared to ten years ago — *nor do patients now, quite frequently, have any great expectations of effective help*. Why is this so?

The first reason is that the shift from more personal care towards technology has undoubtedly in many acute (and indeed potentially fatal) cases achieved amazing results. However, concomitant with this has been the felt loss by many of personal engagement by their doctor with more minor ailments. Patients need human reassurance even if the problem is merely a painful and debilitating boil or a case of chicken-pox, and the disengagement of human with human has meant that they receive this less reliably and less frequently than in the past.

The 'hands of the healer' may be an image that is no longer current, partly because of the fashionably cynical tone of the age. (As a patient, I suspect that many a general practitioner still privately idealises that image, but must hide it from his of her peers.) However, the truth is that in a sick world the 'hands of healing' (in a deeper and wider sense than mere technology) are a human need, because the 'hands' are human. Thus there is a huge gap between what it is possible to say to our doctors we want, and what we most deeply want. Even the sacred goal of curtailing waiting times may be achieved at too high a cost.

Consider, for instance, the ambiguous 'good' of some near-production-line medicine, where a general practitioner can refer patients to the cardiac department of a rapid diagnosis clinic: 'There they are examined by a process which leaves them untouched by human hand. They pass from one examination to another, very often without seeing a doctor'.[3] 'Surely', my friend Dr J said to me, 'it's better for the patient to have someone who is technically excellent, even if they're no good at the "personal care" bit.' To which the vast majority of patients would reply that this is a non-question, because for no doctor should this be a choice, and it is a failure of medical practice if it is. The patient's whole humanness is as crucial to the diagnostic and treatment process as is that of the general practitioner – and it must be recovered. In other words, *we look for the rehumanisation of the patient.*

What Alder Hey has taught us

Although the issue of Alder Hey's use of babies' body parts was a hospital matter, not an issue of primary care, it nevertheless focuses in an excellent manner an issue which runs right through our medical services. In rightly seeking to further medical technology, those involved at the hospital forgot one thing that was needful, indeed all-important – they were still dealing with human beings. The Bishop of Liverpool identified this memorably at the Alder Hey memorial service:

> This is why the taking of our children's organs and tissues has been such an offence to parents and families. When your child is sick and helpless, you hold them to yourself to let them feel the warmth and reassurance of your body. When they die, the memory you cherish is the warmth of that embrace – body to body, flesh to flesh, heart to heart. The body – *their* body – weak and vulnerable, pressed against yours – strong and caring – hoping for a miracle. ... To discover that their body – so precious to your memory – has been violated leaves you understandably traumatised. Their body and the memory of their body are both marred. ... When you discover what has been done without your knowledge, without your understanding, without your consent, you feel betrayed – *so much so that it becomes difficult to trust anybody in authority.*[4]

The truth is that doctors, having fought back from dehumanisation, are now – in the public perception – in many ways all too human. The public 'death of deference' has been adjudged healthy and good by some general practitioners. However, 'deference' is a very different quality from 'respect', and it is the latter which needs to be recovered on both sides in the doctor–patient relationship. The roundedness of the humanity of the general practitioner is a perception that patients *owe* to their doctors, but this can only be achieved if general practitioners also give back to their patients *their* humanness – and each can start by giving the other the dignity of respect.

Appraisals and sanctions

The public recognition of the human fallibility of doctors has seen the putting in place of robust mechanisms to check the reliability of the service offered. However, here we encounter the very difficulty that Baroness O'Neill raised in her probing Reith Lectures on the nature of 'trust'. Trust in the medical profession cannot be achieved by means of fail-safe mechanisms, because then we patients are trusting not the doctor but the checks and balances, the fail-safe mechanisms, which are appraising and checking that doctor. At best it leads not to a relationship of human with human – the necessity that I have been urging – but rather to a legalistic relationship of client with service agency, defined and lived out by contract rather than by commitment – a sort of *mélange* of consumerism and legalism. To quote Baroness O'Neill:

> The common ground from which I begin is that we cannot have guarantees that everyone will keep trust. Elaborate measures to ensure that people keep agreements and do not betray trust must, in the end, be backed by – trust. There is, I think, no complete answer to the old question, 'Who will guard the guardians?'. On the contrary, trust is needed because all guarantees are incomplete. Guarantees are useless unless they lead to a trusted source, and a regress of guarantees is no better for being longer unless it ends in a trusted source. So trust cannot presuppose or require a watertight guarantee of others' performance, and cannot rationally be withheld just because we lack guarantees. Where we have guarantees or proofs, we don't need trust. ... So we take elaborate steps to deter and prevent deception and fraud: we set and enforce high standards. ... Contracts clarify and formalise agreements and undertakings with ever greater precision. Professional codes define professional responsibilities with ever greater accuracy.[5]

The point, of course, is that *contracts* are based on the assumption that trust can fail. Therefore their basis is always that worst-case scenario – the betrayal of trust – hence their minatory tone and legalistic approach to the inevitabilities of human failure. Equally inevitably, this colours the doctor–patient relationship.

Accepting honest failure:
the patient's responsibility

Few of us ordinary patients instinctively put our trust in *systems* rather than in *persons*, so the current attempt to transfer the relationship of trust to the system is to ignore a simple psychological fact. And where there is also – as there is felt to have been – *systemic* failure, the non-trust is compounded. The latter is not helped by the public sense that doctors have tended to combine together to present a common front against systemic change, reform or criticism. The recent scandals have deepened this conviction – in the identified 'cover-ups', or at best the ignoring of observable medical malpractice.

But *why* has there been this professional closing of ranks – even to the extent of obscuring of an objective appraisal of the facts in any one incident? Here we patients must accept our own share of responsibility, and recognise that clamouring for harsh sanctions and an over-rigorous approach may well be counter-productive – not only to our own interest as patients, but to any setting right of errors arising from either system or individual. Liam Donaldson, the Government's Chief Medical Officer, identified this tellingly after, as he said, being involved with the Cleveland child abuse crisis, the Bristol children's heart surgery case, the Alder Hey affair and, as Chief Medical Officer, the case of Dr Harold Shipman. He had concluded that:

> You can only regain trust if first of all there's openness on the part of those providing public services, but also a willingness to admit failure. And the problem is that an admission of failure these days is usually met with the reaction of blame and retribution. So … is it possible to regain trust without a greater public understanding that there is such a thing as honest failure? Is it possible, unless we can avoid accountability always being mediated through blame and retribution?[6]

What he was pointing to was the fact that a doctor who is prepared to admit mistakes is likely to be an honest doctor and therefore deserving of *trust*. However, if our general practitioners are constantly battered by sanctions on behalf of us patients, and often faced with a demand for compensation if any fault is admitted, we then re-enter the legalistic client–server consumerist contractual relationship which excludes 'trust' and relies on penalties. As a patient I see this clearly, and therefore strongly support the aim of current complaint procedures which remove the 'blame' factor unless the issue is so serious as to be formalised. I would want my doctor to know that he can admit failure without losing my trust, and certainly without my prosecuting him.

Politicisation of medical practice

As if the sense of being shifted to a lawyer–client relationship were not destructive enough of trust, the last two decades of politicisation of medicine in the public perception have added another layer of non-trust. One obvious example was the public anxiety over the MMR vaccine.

The suspicion which surrounded the MMR vaccine was greatly increased when the Government was seen to be pressing for its use. Thus we patients had to struggle not only with the difficulties that I have outlined, and therefore a somewhat guarded *non*-trusting legalistic view of our general practitioner's advice, but also with our own widespread and profound *mis*trust of politicians, particularly if they happen to be in Government. As patients we found ourselves weighing the issue of MMR with huge anxiety. My godchild, a former ward sister who is now the mother of a child of vaccinable age, was even *more* confused as to the right thing to do (medically informed as she was), because of *Government* pressure in the debate, than she had been by the advice of her doctor.

A major reason for mistrusting advice is that we patients know of the financial inducements to general practitioners to advocate specific treatments or diagnostic processes (e.g. the cervical smear), so *of course* it is harder for us to trust the objectivity of the doctor's opinion. In *The Guardian*'s very interesting Special

Report on the general practitioner service (published in August 2002), there was one doctor who spoke, it seems to me, for all patients as well as for all general practitioners when he said that he 'had no doubt that the success of his work depended upon the creation of a bond of trust that binds him to his patients. Therefore they must not suspect him of prescribing to protect his salary.'[7]

NICE: a solution or a smokescreen?

The Government's medicines watchdog, the National Institute for Clinical Excellence (NICE), was set up in an attempt publicly to distance difficult decision making about the prescribing of expensive treatments from the individual general practitioner, the local primary healthcare trust, the Government itself and the 'postcode lottery' in general. However, because of the politicisation of medicine, it has been seen by some as a smokescreen, concealing advice or pressure from the Government behind the scenes. So its latest attempt to become more trusted has been to create a 'Citizens' Council', recruiting 50 members of the public to assemble for two three-day meetings a year to look at some of the issues facing NICE, and to give their views. This is particularly crucial in those areas which raise ideological or ethical questions (e.g. whether scarce medical funds should be used to treat conditions that are lifestyle oriented, such as smoking or obesity).

For it is clear that one of the profound problems that bedevils the practice of medicine and leads to the further erosion of doctor–patient trust is that there is no public consensus and no official Government policy on such ideological questions – hence an attempt to take a public 'sounding'. However, the chorus of cynical comment which has greeted this proposal shows how difficult it is to achieve accepted trustworthiness in a climate of political suspicion. For instance, Liam Fox, Shadow Health Secretary, described it (predictably) as a 'second fig-leaf' that the Government was adding to the first fig-leaf of NICE itself: 'The Government has undermined NICE since the day it was created. The Government forced NICE to consider not just whether a drug was cost-effective, but whether it was affordable in the first place – a job politicians should be accountable for'.

The distinction between cost-effectiveness and affordability is a real one, and such accusations need a public answer. However, such reactions also highlight how difficult it is for the patient to do anything other than develop a suspicion that even a move such as this – seeking the advice of a Citizens' Council – may not be trustworthy. No wonder the poor general practitioner feels the fallout!

The paradox of progress

Thus as a patient I have to face the fact that all of the 'improvements' or safeguards in the process of primary care which I have demanded – a reduction in waiting times, monitoring of the quality of medical services, geographical equity in prescribing, separation of Government from prescription assessment, 'justice' when things go wrong – are, of necessity and paradoxically, the cause of further non-trust, through the distancing that they create between my general practitioner and me. With Onora O'Neill I recognise the difference between accountability and trust, and the counter-productive effects of stressing the former to the detriment of the latter. With the general practitioners I recognise that I have in the past 'dehumanised' them, as they have since 'dehumanised' me, and that I must therefore seek means to return the human dimension to my perception of my general practitioner (as he must to me). What does this mean in practice?

1   It means being prepared to pay more in taxes, *and telling the Government so*, to enable a huge increase in the number of general practitioners, so that with more time for each patient, each doctor can develop the skills of humanity.
2   It means working to establish a culture in which the general practitioner can admit a mistake without peremptory loss of the professional relationship of trust between doctor and patient.
3   It means that I, too, as a patient must remove the 'mechanistic' from our relationship. I must not see my doctor primarily as the assured technological answer to all my ills, but as a fellow human being, struggling in a battle that never ceases against sickness and mortality – a battle which I am sharing with him in my own body.
4   Further to this, it means recognising, when we meet in the consulting room, that this is someone with his own load in which I could at least show interest. (At the most basic level, how many of us as patients ask our doctor how *he* is before expanding on our own needs?)

And how might the general practitioner help?

1   By not losing long-term touch with particular patients. 'Diagnosing by telephone is easy', said Dr S, *'if you know the patient'*[7] (my italics). Nothing – not the most detailed of notes – can equal the potential value of personal knowledge built up over the years in the doctor–patient relationship. There are several ways of doing this, through careful organisation of consulting hours and practice.
2   By recognising that, however composed the patient might seem, for most of us *any* visit to the consulting room has an element of stress – we would frankly rather not be there, although we are grateful that we *can* be. For some there is real reluctance and anxiety, although it is often well concealed (after all, we have our pride). But for reasons ranging from a felt sense of invasion of personal privacy to a fear of what the 'judgement' (significant word) of the general practitioner will be, the patient is suffering some tension, however minor the problem and however patient-led the discussion. A good doctor will recognise that this room, which is so familiar to him, is always alien territory to a patient, and will allow for this in the way that he seeks to gain his patient's confidence (*trust*).
3   By taking seriously all available training in 'people skills', and being humble enough to realise that it takes a lifetime to hone them.
4   By so evidently and publicly refusing to succumb to the pressure of 'league-tables' in economic prescribing, or financial gain in promoting some medication or process, that the patient can be sure that the proposed way forward is objectively the best in the general practitioner's view.
5   Finally, by becoming genuinely interested in the patient as a person – and showing it!

Telling the story rather than doing the arithmetic

I suggested earlier that, as patients, our relationship with our general practitioners is currently being shaped by a mixture of legalism and consumerism. In the question and answer session following the third of the Reith Lectures, Onora O'Neill was asked whether, since we live in a market economy based on the measurability of everything (products, costs, and even sanctions), it was not inevitable that professional services such as medicine should be seen as necessarily quantifiable. In reply, O'Neill made a crucial distinction. Indeed, everything could be *called to account*, but it was not always appropriate that the 'account' should be in arithmetical terms – sometimes an account needed to be given in *narrative* rather than arithmetical terms (in story terms rather than in figures).

I believe that as patients and general practitioners it is our common narrative, our shared story, that we need to rediscover, rather than a putative 'value-for-money' estimate in financial or mathematical terms. And I think if each doctor and patient stopped to consider what their common story was, they would again discover each other as mutually respected human beings, and the richness of our professional relationship could be restored.

Perhaps (who knows?) that is the next chapter in our long story. I hope so.

- There appears to be less trust now between general practitioners, their patients and their patients' families than there was in the 1990s.
- The main reason for this is that insufficient attention is being paid to the fundamental importance of the practitioner–patient relationship.
- A professional relationship based on the strong moral qualities of mutual trust and respect seems to be being replaced by a relationship that is based on contract, accountability and the possibility of legal redress.
- The situation is exacerbated by the politicisation of medicine, since patients are inclined to trust doctors but to distrust politicians.
- The key to rebuilding trust is to 'rehumanise' both practitioners and their patients in their relationships with each other.
- Specific changes in attitudes and behaviour on both sides (and from Government) are needed for this to happen.

References

1   Quoted by Roy Hattersley (21 August 2002), 'Special Report on the GP Service', *The Guardian*. Three sequential articles: 'Politics of life in the surgery' (19.8.02); 'Obscure charm of the inner city practice' (20.8.02); 'Creating a new deal for doctors' (21.8.02).
2   Sermon by Bishop James Jones (10 November 2001); copy privately circulated.
3   *The Guardian*, ibid.
4   Bishop James Jones, ibid.
5   Onora O'Neill (13 May 2002), BBC Radio 4, *Reith Lecture 1*. www.bbc.co.uk/radio4/reith2002
6   Question and answer session following the above.
7   Roy Hattersley, ibid.

CHAPTER 2

Trust and mistrust

Rob Innes

Put not your trust in princes, nor in the son of man, in whom there is no help.

(Psalm 146)

Covenants struck without the sword are but words.

(Thomas Hobbes, *Leviathan*)

A nation's well-being ... is conditioned by a single, pervasive cultural char-acteristic: the level of trust.

(Francis Fukuyama)

With a complete absence of trust, one must be catatonic, one could not even get up in the morning.

(Russell Hardin)

This chapter examines the nature of trust. It offers a sociological model of trust, which will be used as a way of evaluating the measures for rebuilding trust that are set out in later chapters of the book.

A culture of suspicion

A whole host of recent high-profile scandals bear witness to an alleged crisis of public trust:

- *in business*: directors of Enron, one of the world's largest oil companies, are found guilty of fraud. What is worse, Enron's auditors, Arthur Andersen, turned a blind eye to false accounting in order not to lose a valued client
- *in politics*: John Major, the 'Mr Clean' of recent British political life, is discovered to have been maintaining an adulterous affair at the time when he launched his 'back to basics' drive on personal morality
- *in the Church*: several North American Roman Catholic dioceses face huge law suits after covering up hundreds of child abuse cases
- *in education*: The 'gold standard' of A-levels has been undermined by alleged interference with grading levels

- and, not least, *in the medical profession*, which has been rocked by poor performance of certain types of heart surgery at Bristol, the widespread retention of children's organs at Alder Hey, and the extraordinary criminal practice of Dr Harold Shipman.

These are simply some of the cases that have hit the headlines. Beyond this there are, some say, deep cultural forces at work which are eroding the bonds of trust. We live in the age of 'late capitalism', 'late modernity' or 'post-modernity'. And this period is characterised by an emphasis on the individual and his or her pleasures and needs. Whereas once we might have derived our identity primarily from our place and status in our community, identity is now increasingly conferred through an acquired 'lifestyle'.

In his book *Lost Icons*,[1] the new Archbishop of Canterbury, Rowan Williams, laments that we are increasingly unable to picture ourselves except through the language of consumer choice. In such a world, other people, even our children, are seen as 'competitors'. Fellowship, charity and trust become increasingly difficult to realise. Likewise, Zygmunt Bauman comments that we have become 'a society which shapes its members first and foremost by the need to play the role of consumer'.[2] And American sociologist Robert Putnam suggests that these corrosive social forces have led to the halving of the available 'social capital' in the USA in the space of four generations.[3]

But have we actually become less trusting? Not according to Onora O'Neill, the Cambridge philosopher and presenter of the 2002 Reith Lectures. She doubts those polls and newspapers which gleefully report declining public trust. The question of trust is, she believes, altogether more complex than is likely to be accurately captured on a pollster's clipboard or in a tabloid newspaper. Our *actions* are, she suggests, a better guide to our true feelings than the things we *say* to the pollsters.

And our actions show that we constantly place trust in others, in members of professions and in public institutions. Nearly all of us drink water supplied by water companies and eat food sold in supermarkets and produced by ordinary farming practices. Nearly all of us use the roads or the trains. Even if we have misgivings, we go on placing trust in the delivery of letters by the Post Office, in the lines maintained by Railtrack, in medicines sold by the pharmaceutical industry and in operations performed in NHS hospitals. 'Where people have options [as they frequently do], we can tell whether they really mistrust by seeing whether they put their money where they put their mouths. The evidence suggests that we still constantly place trust in many of the institutions and professions that we profess not to trust.'[4]

The point made, rather convincingly, by O'Neill is that we do *not* live in a culture of 'mistrust' where individuals refuse to place trust in banks, businesses and hospitals. Rather, we live in a culture of 'suspicion'. Yes, there are *some* untrustworthy politicians, doctors, scientists and businesspeople – but there always have been. And prominent examples of these do not make the case that we are living amid a new or deeper crisis of trust. Rather, the emerging *culture of suspicion* is shown by the degree to which we expect professionals and institutions to demonstrate clearly and convincingly why we should continue to trust them.

However, O'Neill suggests that our suspicious culture is, perversely, generating activities which only serve to make the problem worse. First, there is the widespread and unrealistic assertion of individual 'rights' without a corresponding set of duties. Secondly, there is the whole bureaucratic apparatus of 'accountability', which may end up distorting professional performance so as to meet artificial targets. Thirdly, there is the high value given to a form of 'transparency', which has little to do with uncovering genuine deceit. And fourthly, there has arisen a media culture in which spreading suspicion has become a routine activity.

Have we actually become less trusting, or is it just that we say we are less trusting? This is hard to judge. Whatever answer we give to this question, it is evident that the task of inspiring and sustaining trust is a vital one for all who work as professionals in public institutions. In particular, the doctor–patient relationship depends crucially on trust. And the prevailing culture of suspicion makes the task all the harder. Trust is gained incrementally, but it is lost catastrophically.

Therefore my objective in this chapter is to explore the nature of trust, to set out one particular model of trust, and to suggest within this model how trust between people is built up and maintained.

Trust: the view from theology

Within Christian theology, trust (or faith) is a central concept. Throughout the Bible, the relationship between God and human beings is described principally through the category of faith. It involves three components, namely *notitia* (knowledge of what is to be believed), *assensus* (intellectual acceptance of its truth) and *fiducia* (personal commitment to that truth). Taken as a whole, the Judaeo-Christian tradition does not so much encourage 'blind faith' as 'questioning faith'. Several books of the Hebrew scriptures (Job, Psalms, Ecclesiastes) are concerned with a serious questioning of faith in the face of suffering and meaninglessness. The opposite of faith is not so much questioning and doubt as cynicism and rebellion. Failure to trust a trustworthy God is seen as a sign of human weakness and error.

Historically, there has been a debate as to whether faith (or trust) is a human decision or a divine gift. Is faith an 'active' quality that arises from human understanding and decision (more typically a Catholic view)? Or is it a 'passive' quality that is given by divine grace (more typically a Protestant view)? The same issue arises in human relationships, where trust might be thought to be primarily the decision of the truster, or alternatively it might be thought to be generated mainly by qualities emanating from the trustee.

The Judaeo-Christian scriptures record the activities of a people which believed that its corporate life could be founded on trust. This was expressed in a series of covenants, from Abraham onwards, between the people and their God. It led to a moral and legal system which naturally exalted trustworthiness and denounced falsity and corruption. The first Christian communities were based on a 'new covenant' that embodied a love which 'always protects, always trusts, always hopes, always perseveres'.[5]

Yet although the Judaeo-Christian scriptures by all means encourage trust in God, they are frankly suspicious about the extent to which other human beings, particularly those with political authority, can be trusted. With only a few exceptions, the Old Testament kings are all presented as fundamentally untrustworthy. Even the heroes of the faith are not people one should trust too unquestioningly. For example, Jacob tricks his brother out of his birthright, Joseph sets up his brothers for a theft of silver, King David commits adultery with Bathsheba and murders her husband, and even St Peter cannot be trusted if he is put under pressure.

Trust: the view from philosophy

Much western philosophy shares with strands of Christian theology a sceptical view of human trustworthiness – what we might call the 'X' theory of human nature. Glaucon, in Plato's *Republic*, is an early representative of this position. Glaucon argues that only the fear of detection and punishment prevents a human being from breaking the law and doing evil for the sake of his own self-interest. According to Glaucon's view, we should only trust someone else if we are sure that they fear detection and punishment sufficiently for this to dissuade them from harming or stealing from us. According to this view, I should trust my doctor to prescribe me appropriate treatment – and not, for example, to make me the unknowing guinea pig for a new and untried medicine – only if I think they are sufficiently afraid of being found out and struck off if they do not. Glaucon's position has been continued and developed in the political philosophy of Machiavelli and the social contract theory of Thomas Hobbes – and perhaps by certain Secretaries of State in our own day.

However, Enlightenment philosophers, have taken a rather more optimistic view, what we might call the 'Y' theory of human nature. David Hume, in his *Treatise of Human Nature*, recognises that among the basic human sentiments are a degree of love and sympathy which makes for more trust – even between princes – than Machiavelli or Hobbes would allow. Hume believed that increasing civilisation and education would tend to increase the level of human fellow-feeling and trust. John Locke and Immanuel Kant argued that we share an innate sense of morality which could be cultivated in order to overcome our tendencies to self-interest. According to this more positive view, we trust others because we believe in their natural love, sympathy and morality. Thus I trust my doctor because I believe (in the absence of strong evidence to the contrary) that she is a good person who cares for my welfare.

Although there is probably a measure of truth in both the 'X' and 'Y' theories, I do not consider that either of them is really adequate. The patient can surely be expected to place trust in the doctor neither solely because of the doctor's fear of detection for malpractice nor solely because of the doctor's feelings of sympathy or their moral sense. The 'X' theory generates a culture of blame and punishment, which will only serve to erode whatever benevolence the doctor might possess. On the other hand, the 'Y' theory seems to promote a hope which risks being severely disappointed. Perhaps a more adequate, rational basis for trust may derive from the notion that human beings, doctors included, are the kind of beings who have the ability to *take responsibility* for others.[6]

It is reasonable to trust my doctor if I believe that he or she has taken responsibility for my health and is competent to exercise this responsibility. In this case I may even, under certain circumstances, feel that it is right to hand over decision making about my health to the doctor. For it is in fact this 'taking of responsibility' which is the essence of professional life and conduct. The ability to 'take responsibility' comes close to the heart of what we typically understand as growth into mature human adulthood. It makes sense to trust if one believes (as seems at least plausible, and at best obvious) that human beings are the kind of creatures that can and will, under certain conditions, take responsibility. The social task of fostering trust is then a matter of creating those conditions in society that are conducive to the proper taking and exercising of such professional responsibility.

At this point, the philosopher needs to hand over to the sociologist. For we must ask what kinds of conditions in society make for responsible, trustworthy individuals and institutions.

Trust: the view from sociology

As it happens, the question of how to build and sustain trust within society has, in the last decade, moved to centre stage within the social sciences. Thus the sociologist Barbara Misztal writes that 'The questions of how social trust is produced and what kinds of social trust enhance economic and governmental performance increasingly become the central set of theoretical issues in social sciences.'[7] Within the political realm, the renewal of civil society has become a basic part of the 'Third Way' espoused by Tony Blair and theoretised by Anthony Giddens.[8] And at the centre of the idea of civil society are questions about mutual responsibility and trust.

There is therefore a considerable volume of recent sociological writing on the question of trust. One of the most significant recent sociological treatises in the area is that by the Polish Professor of Sociology (now based at Cambridge University), Piotr Sztompka.[9] Sztompka builds on previous work by, for example, Luhmann,[10] Misztal,[7] Gambetta,[11] Giddens[12] and Fukuyama.[13] He offers a comprehensive theory of trust, and provides a model to explain how 'trust cultures' rise (and fall). The work has particular authenticity because of the author's own experience of the effects of the absence of trust in his native Poland, and his analysis of the attempts to rebuild trust after the collapse of communism.

In the remaining sections of this chapter I shall give an outline of Sztompka's theory, which will provide a framework for locating the practical suggestions for building trust in healthcare that are offered in the central section of this book.

Sztompka's model of trust

Sztompka puts forward many reasons why the problem of trust has become prominent in contemporary societies. Among them are the following.

1   He shares with Luhmann and Giddens the idea that we have moved from a society based on fate to a risk-based society. The suggestion is that the degree to which human beings have been able to influence and control their own futures has varied greatly over the course of history. We no longer face the future dependent upon fortune or providence. Rather, we plan and make calculated decisions about the future, and we place our trust in the outcome of these decisions.
2   Our world has become increasingly interdependent through, for example, market forces and globalisation.

3   Large sections of the contemporary world have become opaque for their members. More often than previously we have to act in the dark. Without trust we would be paralysed and unable to act.
4   Those upon whom we depend are increasingly anonymous to us.
5   The technological world that we have created carries the possibility of disastrous failure.
6   In all areas of life we have more choice, and therefore there is less predictability. Trust becomes more salient for our decisions and our actions as the feasible set of alternatives that are open to us becomes larger.

For Sztompka, therefore, trust is an active choice, against passive acceptance of fate. It is concerned with leaving the discourse of fate and entering the discourse of agency. 'Trust is a bet about the future contingent actions of others.'[14] Because my decision to trust – having weighed up the evidence – is my decision, then I alone am responsible for the outcome. 'Because in this case, we actively commit ourselves, we can no longer blame others, nor the regime, nor the system, if something goes wrong.'[15]

Recalling our theological analysis of faith, it is evident that Sztompka's account embodies the three components of *notitia* (knowledge of what is to be believed), *assensus* (intellectual acceptance of its truth) and *fiducia* (personal commitment to that truth). However, what it firmly rules out is the 'passive' dimension of faith. Sztompka's trust is a thoroughly 'active' quality.

This, I think, is a weakness of the theory (although not a disastrous weakness). Stzompka makes a sharp distinction between 'trust', which he thinks is an active quality, and 'confidence', which is a passive quality. However, in practice these categories overlap. Most of us (including the *Oxford English Dictionary*) consider that trust includes an element of 'confidence' in someone or something, which is not necessarily an 'active' quality. This applies especially in situations where we are weak – as the recipients of medical care typically are. The elderly patient lying in a hospital bed does not usually run through various future scenarios, calculate the risks, decide whether to trust, and then accept sole responsibility for the outcome. Indeed, the very word 'patient' (if we are allowed to use it instead of 'customer') is linked etymologically to being 'passive'.

Notwithstanding this reservation, I believe that Sztompka's subsequent theory covering the varieties of and foundations for trust is extremely valuable. He distinguishes three types of trust, namely personal, positional and institutional, and he argues that these are all linked in complex ways. For example, 'If trust attaches to a certain social role (position) then it extends to every incumbent. But the personal trust vested in incumbents is not irrelevant for preserving, enhancing or diminishing positional trust, and even converting itself into trust for the whole institution.'[16] Thus trust in doctors could convert itself into trust in the NHS. However, Sztompka also notices that there are situations where trust does not carry over from institutions to positions. For example, one might trust 'democracy' but not trust 'politicians'. It is therefore important to unravel exactly where trust and mistrust lie. Do they lie in individual nurses and doctors? Or in the professions? Or in the institutions of the NHS?

Sztompka further notices that trust means 'A trusts B to do X'. Trust is not completely open-ended. So we have to ask 'what kind of trust?'. For example, in the case of doctors, he quotes a survey which shows that:

Table 2.1   Sztompka's model of trust

Primary trust	Reputation	Track record and status of the professional person and occupational group
	Performance	Present experience with this person
	Appearance	Subjective impact of people and buildings
Secondary trust	Accountability	Existence (or not) of a credible enforcement regime
	Pre-commitment	Willingness of the professional to go beyond normal contractual requirements
	Situation	Social setting (intimate and local or anonymous)
Trusting impulse		The client's psychological propensity to trust
Trust culture		The norms and values in the wider society that favour or militate against trust

1   82% of people expect their doctor to be competent
2   60% of people expect their doctor to be sympathetic and helpful.

Thus a doctor might breach a patient's trust in one of two very different ways. Neither the technically competent but brusque doctor nor the nice but ineffectual doctor meet the full range of patient needs. To be sure that a doctor is fully 'trusted', we would have to identify all of the main qualities in which the patient has invested expectations.

So, given that trust is a multi-dimensional category, how do we set about building it? Sztompka identifies four 'foundations' of trust, which he calls primary trust, secondary trust, the trusting impulse and the trust culture (*see* Table 2.1). I shall briefly discuss each of these in turn.

Primary trust

The most important ground for trust is the truster's estimate of the trustworthiness of the target on which they are considering bestowing their trust. Sztompka calls this *primary trust*. Primary trust refers to those traits and qualities of the person or institution which make them worthy of trust. Sztompka identifies three bases of primary trust.

1   *Reputation*: this is established by such factors as a person's track record, their qualifications, second-hand testimonies and stories, and the personal experience of the truster. Reputation is a valuable personal and professional asset.

2   *Performance*: this refers to actual deeds, present conduct and currently obtained results. The past is suspended, and we focus on how the candidate for our trust is doing now.

3   *Appearance*: trust may be evoked (or diminished) by a whole range of external features (e.g. physiognomy, body language, intonation, readiness to smile, dress, age, race, gender). All institutions are made manifest by the 'agents' who work as their public face, and their appearance matters. However, the appearance of buildings themselves can also create or erode institutional trust.

Secondary trust

The trustworthiness of people and institutions may be due not only to their immanent qualities (reputation, performance and appearance), but also to the context and environment in which their actions take place. Sztompka identifies three types of contextual conditions that are most relevant for enhancing trustworthiness.

1   *Accountability*: the enforcement of trustworthiness, in particular through the presence of agencies that monitor and sanction the conduct of the trustee. As Machiavelli and Hobbes realised, I am more likely to trust someone if I know it is also in their interests to prove trustworthy.

2   *Pre-commitment*: this refers to a situation where the parties take on some extra commitment or obligation, beyond what is normally required, which functions as an additional demonstration of trust. The example that Stzompka majors on is American 'covenant marriage', in which the partners voluntarily renounce the right to a no-fault divorce, as a demonstration of their mutual commitment and trust in each other.

3   *Situation*: groups where people know each other well in different settings, groups that share high moral codes, tightly knit communities, and encounters in sacred or quasi-sacred settings all tend to increase trust.

The trusting impulse

There are certain psychological factors which predispose some people to be more trusting than others. Sztompka refers to a 'trusting impulse' that is derived from early experiences in life. Children learn to be trusting adults, he suggests, through positive experiences of home and family life. There may be a 'universal impulse towards sociability' which needs to be nurtured and developed. Thus building trust is not just a matter of having trustworthy people and institutions – it is also a matter of forming people who are capable of placing trust. Based on his experience in Poland, Sztompka suggests that this involves such things as fostering strong family life, encouraging trusting relationships in schools, openness to religious insights, and encouraging public discourse about moral choice.

Trust culture

In the same way as the trusting impulse is a product of personal biography, so we may speak of a 'trust culture' which is the product of institutional or national history. Cultures grow 'from below' out of the countless small choices of ordinary people. They are also directed 'from above' by the personalities and policies of politicians, leaders and visionaries. In effect, culture acquires certain persisting, lasting qualities that embody the institution's collective memory. Culture is made known through values, norms, symbols, patterns of discourse, and so on.

In Sztompka's terms, a 'trust culture' is a system of norms and values that regulate, grant, meet, return and reciprocate trust. Trust culture accumulates and codifies rules about trust and trustworthiness into prevailing, lasting experiences with various types of trust. Sztompka recalls how, in communist Poland, it was regarded as appropriate to trust people in the private domain, but generally inappropriate to trust people in the public domain. Yet even within the latter, some institutions were to be trusted more than others. For example, the army was to be trusted much more than the police, and the parliament was to be trusted more than the communist party.

A trust culture exerts pressure on people to make choices in certain kinds of ways. Positive, trusting 'bets on the future' are much more unlikely to occur if the culture discourages them.

Stzompka offers a valuable model of trust. Although we do not follow it slavishly in this book, we do commend it as a useful framework for thinking about the issues. In the chapters that follow we shall look at how trust has been eroded within the health service. We shall then consider a raft of proposals for rebuilding trust. In the concluding chapters, we shall return to Stzompka to consider how adequately his different 'bases of trust' have been addressed.

- We live in a culture that encourages us to be suspicious of others, especially those in authority.
- Such a culture tends to generate 'controls' on people that only make us more suspicious.
- Professionals need to find ways of demonstrating trustworthiness that are genuinely effective.
- Trust involves confidence, but it is more than confidence.
- We shall not find a solution to the problem if we assume that people are wholly self-interested ('X theory') or wholly benevolent ('Y theory').
- It is better to look at the social conditions which generate trustworthy people and institutions.
- According to Sztompka's model of trust, we need to build primary trust, secondary trust, the trusting impulse and a trust culture.

References

1   Williams R (2000) *Lost Icons*. Continuum, London.
2   Bauman Z (1998) *Work, Consumerism and the New Poor*. Open University Press, Milton Keynes.
3   Putnam R (1995) Bowling alone: America's declining social capital. *J Democracy*. **6**: 65–78.
4   O'Neill O (2002) *Reith Lecture 1*; www.bbc.co.uk/radio4/reith2002.

5   New International Version of the Bible. 1 Corinthians, chapter 13, verse 7.

6   Bailey T (2002) *On Trust and Philosophy*. BBCi Open University; www.open2.net/trust/on_trust/on_trust1.htm

7   Misztal B (1996) *Trust in Modern Societies*. Basil Blackwell, Oxford.

8   Giddens A (1998) *The Third Way*. Polity Press, Cambridge, pp. 78–86.

9   Sztompka P (1999) *Trust: a sociological theory*. Cambridge University Press, Cambridge.

10   Luhmann N (1979) *Trust and Power*. John Wiley & Sons, New York.

11   Gambetta D (ed.) (1988) *Trust: making and breaking co-operative relations*. Basil Blackwell, Oxford.

12   Beck U, Giddens A and Lash S (1994) *Reflexive Modernization*. Polity Press, Cambridge.

13   Fukuyama F (1995) *Trust: the social virtues and creation of prosperity*. Free Press, New York.

14   Sztompka P, op. cit., p. 25.

15   Sztompka P, op. cit., p. 25.

16   Sztompka P, op. cit., p. 48.

CHAPTER 3

The Shipman case: the individual

Richard Baker

I wish all general practitioners could have stood in front of that audience, and breathed in the smell of trust betrayed, and understood and accepted the duty now placed on us.

(Richard Baker)

This chapter chronicles Shipman's killing behaviour, and argues that uncertainty about systems of prevention and detection is more appropriate than uncertainty about the medical profession as a whole. Nevertheless, doctors do need to appraise the systems which monitor and regulate their profession.

In her first report, Dame Janet Smith, Chairman of the Shipman Inquiry, wrote:

> Shipman has also damaged the good name of the medical profession and has caused many patients to doubt whether they can trust their own family doctor. This trust forms the relationship between doctor and patient. Although I believe that the overwhelming majority of patients will, on reflection, realise that they can indeed trust their doctor as they always have done, there will be some who remain uncertain.[1]

Is the uncertainty among some patients justified? And how should doctors (in this case, general practitioners) and health service policy makers respond? This chapter will address these questions. First, I shall argue that uncertainty about the systems for preventing or detecting malicious behaviour by general practitioners is more justified than uncertainty about the profession of general practice as a whole. Secondly, I shall argue that the response of the profession should be to review and press for appropriate changes to existing prevention and detection systems.

The detailed accounts of Shipman's activities have appeared in publications which are not readily accessible. Most people have relied on press reports. This chapter therefore begins with a summary of the salient points based on my own review of his clinical practice[2] and the Shipman Inquiry's first report.[1] This is followed by a discussion of the implications for patient trust, and a presentation of the two arguments.

A history of murder

Harold Frederick Shipman (known as Fred) was born in 1946. He was admitted to Leeds University Medical School in 1965, and gained provisional registration with the General Medical Council (GMC) in July 1970. After pre-registration house jobs in Pontefract, and subsequent junior hospital posts, he was appointed initially as assistant general practitioner by the partners of Todmorden Group Practice in Todmorden, West Yorkshire, in 1974. Within a few weeks he became a principal in general practice, but by September 1975 Shipman had left the practice. It was discovered that he had been unlawfully obtaining pethidine and using the drug himself. He pleaded guilty at Halifax Magistrates Court to three offences of obtaining pethidine by deception, three offences of unlawful possession of pethidine and two offences of forgery of an NHS prescription, and he asked for 74 similar offences to be taken into account. He was fined, and the matter was subsequently considered by the GMC, as a result of which Shipman was issued with a warning.

In 1977 he returned to general practice, joining the Donneybrook House Group Practice in Hyde, Greater Manchester, but in 1992 he moved to a single-handed practice in Hyde, retaining his list of registered patients. In September 1998 he was arrested, and in January 2000 he was convicted of the murder of 15 of his older female patients, and of forging the will of one.

The review of his clinical practice and the Inquiry reached very similar conclusions about the number of killings. However, it should, be noted that the review was concerned with analyses of the excess numbers of deaths and whether information in records and cremation forms raised concern about the true cause of death. The Inquiry, on the other hand, undertook a detailed case-by-case investigation drawing on all available sources of evidence, including witness statements, and reached a decision on whether the death of each of Shipman's patients had been natural or unlawful. The conclusion of the review was that the excess number of deaths about which there should be concern was 236 (95% confidence interval: 198–277). The Inquiry considered 888 cases, giving a written decision in 494 cases, and in the remaining 394 cases there was compelling evidence that Shipman was not involved. The Inquiry found that Shipman killed 215 patients (the first in March 1975 and the last in June 1998). In an additional 45 cases, the Inquiry found real suspicion that Shipman may have been responsible, although the evidence was not sufficiently clear for a positive conclusion to be reached.

The progression of Shipman's killings is illustrated in Figure 3.1, which shows the cumulative total numbers of excess deaths from 1974 to 1998 among people dying at home or on practice premises. Key points in Shipman's career and selected information about the killings as determined by the Inquiry are shown in Table 3.1. After the break in his career from 1975 to 1977, he returned to killing in 1978, less than a year after joining the group practice in Hyde. He continued to kill throughout the 1980s, but for some reason in 1990 and 1991 the killings almost ceased. Dame Janet Smith, in the first report of the Inquiry, noted that in November 1989 Shipman only narrowly avoided being caught by the district nurse in the act of killing a patient. Since the circumstances would have prompted some discussion within the practice, this experience may have caused him to suppress his killing behaviour until he could move to the single-handed practice. Following transfer to this practice, the pattern of killing recurred, and the Inquiry classed 16 deaths in 1993 as unlawful, and two more as suspicious. Thereafter the

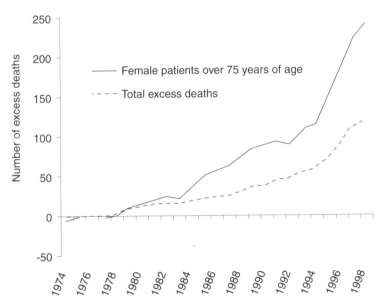

Figure 3.1   Cumulative number of excess deaths caused by Shipman among patients dying at home or on practice premises, as estimated in the review.[2]

killings continued unabated, and in 1997 the total number of people definitely killed during the year was an incredible 37.

Certain features are associated with Shipman's killings. The most common victims were women aged 75 years or over, and the oldest victim was aged 93 years. However, younger women were also killed, as were some men, the youngest victim being a 41-year-old man with terminal illness. Typically, killings took place in the victim's own home, although they also occurred on practice premises, and three killings took place in residential or nursing homes. The most common (but not exclusive) time of day for the killings was the afternoon, and they were less common at weekends. Shipman usually used intravenous diamorphine to kill patients, and gave a plausible cause of death on the death certificate, often supported by fabricated clinical histories and false information recorded on cremation certificates. He took care to avoid the referral of the deaths of his victims to the coroner.

Perhaps to help to reduce the risk of detection, Shipman took care to create for himself a reputation as an 'old-fashioned' doctor – one who would care for his patients at home rather than admit them to hospital, and who would willingly visit them at home, often calling on them unannounced. The motive for Shipman's killings is unclear, and Dame Janet Smith concluded that the explanation lay within his personality, although the detailed factors at work cannot be determined with confidence.[1]

System failure or failure of the profession?

How should the medical profession, and general practitioners in particular, respond to the revelations of Shipman's crimes in order to regain the trust of those patients who remain 'uncertain'? Published responses to date have three elements. First,

Table 3.1 Key points in Shipman's general practice career, and selected information about the numbers of unlawful killings as determined by the Shipman Inquiry[1]

GP in Todmorden	Drug offences	1977: October, joins group practice in Hyde			Sets up single-handed practice in Hyde, with same list of patients, in January 1992		1996: 30 unlawful killings	1998: March, brief police investigation draws a blank.; July, forged a will; September, arrested
1975: March, first unlawful killing	1977: clinical medical officer, South West Durham	1978: August, first unlawful killing in Hyde	1984–89: unlawful killings during the year, and another 4 suspicious deaths	1988: 11 unlawful killings	1990–92: only 3 unlawful killings during this period	1995: 29 unlawful killings		1997: 37 unlawful killings

criticism of all general practitioners would be inappropriate. Secondly, some systems appear to have failed and therefore need review. Thirdly, a determined and enterprising killer could probably defeat any conceivable system. It has been argued that Shipman was unique, and that there is little to be learned about general practice or its governance from his behaviour.[3–5] From this perspective, Shipman's case can be regarded as a breach of trust by an individual, but the breach does not extend to other general practitioners or to the medical profession as a whole. The extension to all general practitioners of the search for an explanation as to why Shipman was able to be so prolific a killer yet escape detection would be fruitless. It could also be harmful, by leading to unjustified criticism of general practitioners, and their consequent alienation.[6]

Others have argued that the response should concentrate on the investigation and possible reform of systems that failed to detect Shipman at an early stage.[7–9] Such systems include cremation certification, referral of deaths to the coroner when the cause of death is uncertain, and the review of prescribing of controlled drugs. Yet even if these systems were reformed, the detection of a future serial killer could not be guaranteed. A determined and devious killer would use all kinds of tactics to avoid detection. One of the implications of the acceptance that system failure was one factor in the failure to detect Shipman is that the breach of trust was not merely individual, but also organisational. The health service failed to operate procedures to protect patients from unlawful killing. In order to regain trust, system reform is required.

The review of Shipman's clinical practice concluded with seven recommendations (see Box 3.1). These are concerned with systems, and are based on the premise that the systems in place at that time had proved inadequate. This view is reiterated in the Inquiry's first report. For example:

> The procedures for certifying and registering deaths – and, in particular, those for obtaining authority to cremate – are intended to provide some safeguard for the public against concealment of the fact that a person has been unlawfully killed. However, even with those procedures in place, I have found that Shipman was able to kill 215 people over a period of 23 years. It is clear, therefore, that the existing procedures provided no safeguard at all, either because they were flawed in themselves, or because they were not properly implemented or, possibly, by reason of a combination of these factors.[1]

Box 3.1   Recommendations made in the review of Shipman's clinical practice

1   Systems for the monitoring of general practitioners should be reviewed and extended to include routine monitoring of death rates, and improved methods for the reveiew of prescribing of controlled drugs and the quality of medical records.

2   A system for collecting information about the numbers of deaths of patients of general practitioners, and the numbers of medical certificates of cause of death issued by general practitioners, should be investigated and a practical system introduced as soon as possible.

3 In a revised certification system, brief information about the circumstances of death and the patient's clinical history should be recorded in the case of both cremations and burials.

4 The procedure for the revalidation of general practitioners should inlcude an assessment of appropriate samples of a general practitioner's records.

5 The policy of offering to return records to general practitioners after the expiry of the required period of storage by health authorities should be reviewed. If general practitioners are allowed to retain records, arrangements for their secure storage should be established, and provision for their eventual disposal agreed.

6 An effective system for the inspection of general practitioners' controlled drugs registers should be introduced.

7 General practitioners should record batch numbers in clinical records when they personally administer controlled drugs, and batch numbers should be included in the controlled drugs registers of general practitioners and pharmacists.

An audit of the accuracy of cremation certificates has confirmed that not only general practitioners but also hospital consultants and junior doctors frequently make errors in completing the certificates.[10] Of 835 sets of forms, only 345 (41%) were completed sufficiently accurately for cremation to proceed without further enquiry. The authors of this audit concluded that the overhaul of existing procedures was long overdue, but also thought that their findings indicated a general belief among doctors that death certification is not a particularly important task. Thus, at least with regard to cremation certification procedures, Dame Janet Smith's report is supported by evidence independent of Shipman.

There is also reason to question the procedures for monitoring the prescribing of controlled drugs. The Regional Medical Service, established in 1920, used to have the task of informing doctors of their obligations under the Misuse of Drugs Act, including the maintenance of controlled drugs registers.[11] However, the Regional Medical Service was disbanded as part of the 1990 NHS reforms, and the fragmented system that replaced it did not uncover Shipman's illicit use of diamorphine. A survey of controlled drug procedures in general practices in one health district confirmed that there were weaknesses in the recording and disposal of drugs.[12] It is therefore reasonable to conclude that a breach of trust by an individual, if sufficiently heinous, can generate questions about the trustworthiness of the healthcare organisation and its systems. The uncertainty of some patients about the systems appears to be justified.

The individual and the organisation

The preceding discussion suggests a distinction between trust in the individual and trust in the organisation and its systems. This distinction has been noted by others.[13,14] Thus it is possible for a patient to lose trust in the systems that regulate doctors but still trust their own general practitioner. With regard to the individual doctor, trust is a recursive feature of the doctor–patient relationship. Through his or her assessment of a doctor's behaviour, the patient develops a degree of trust, and is more likely to develop a continuing relationship with that doctor, thus giving rise to further opportunities for trust to develop in future consultations. When deciding whether a doctor can be trusted, the patient attaches considerable weight to the doctor's behaviour[15] rather than any objective assessment of competence. For example, among patients attending general practitioners there is an association between longitudinal continuity, trust and satisfaction with consultations.[16,17] Increasing continuity is associated with increased trust in the doctor, and if patients consult the doctor they trust, levels of satisfaction are high. In contrast, if patients do not have high levels of trust in their doctor, continuity does not increase satisfaction, and discontinuity does not reduce it.

Since patients cannot make detailed assessments of the competence of their doctors, healthcare organisations, including regulatory systems, are obliged to do what they can to ensure that the patient's *assumption* about the doctor's trustworthiness is not misplaced. Policies on the funding of services such as GP fund-holding, incentives for reaching immunisation targets, or managed care systems[18] may have an impact on patients' views on whether they can trust the healthcare system and even their own doctor. Policies specifically concerned with the competence and performance of doctors might counteract such uncertainty. Such policies are usually expressed in regulatory and monitoring systems. These are intended to detect or prevent extremely serious misconduct or poor performance. In the cases of Shipman, Green (the Loughborough GP paedophile), Ledward and Neale (the Kent and Yorkshire gynaecologists, respectively, who were eventually struck off for malpractice), the systems appear to have failed. They must inevitably be reviewed.

Could it have been different?

What opportunities were presented to the regulatory and monitoring systems with regard to Shipman? They include the following.

- The General Medical Council's review in 1976 following Shipman's conviction for drug offences resulted in Shipman being told that if he offended again, the cases would form part of a subsequent hearing. However, he was allowed to continue in practice unsupervised. At the time the health service did not have any system in place to ensure that managers were aware of the drug offences.
- There were complaints made against Shipman in 1985, 1989, 1992 and 1995. However, no systematic investigation of his performance appears to have been undertaken.
- The health service did not have a system for monitoring mortality rates in general practice, nor were there any systems for the periodic objective assessment of doctors' continued fitness to practise.

However, these opportunities cannot be regarded as failures, as a detailed investigation into each has yet to be completed. Reasonable explanations may emerge. Nevertheless, they do raise the possibility that the profession's regulatory and monitoring systems were inadequate.

To return to the first question posed at the beginning of this chapter, should patients remain uncertain about the trustworthiness of general practitioners? The answer is that although there has been a brutal betrayal of trust by Shipman, exacerbated by system failure, the assumption of a failure on the part of the profession of general practice would be premature. This individual failure of trust should not cause the patient to be uncertain about the trustworthiness of every individual general practitioner. The Inquiry has yet to consider the broader questions relating to general practice, and until that review has been completed, the role of the profession's structures, policies and habits cannot be fully assessed. The list of issues that the Inquiry plans to address in stage four of its deliberations (*see* Box 3.2) provides some clues as to what might be relevant. It would be unwise to speculate on what the conclusions might be, since the Inquiry still has much work to do. In contrast, there are good reasons to believe that there were system failures, and any response to Shipman's crimes must include review and reform of the systems that failed.

Box 3.2 General issues relating to general practice to be considered by the inquiry

- Whistleblowing.
- The systems for monitoring or analysing mortality rates. What did such systems reveal about Shipman?
- The system for monitoring the performance of general medical practitioners, with particular reference to those in single-person practice, record keeping and prescribing.
- Disciplinary rules for general medical practitioners, and the disciplinary processes operated within the NHS and by the General Medical Council. Powers of suspension.
- What information is recorded that arises from errors and complaints?
- The role of patients and their complaints in the monitoring of a GP's practice.
- The role of practice staff in reporting on the performance of a GP.
- How was Shipman's work monitored and with what result?
- The accountability of GPs and health authorities.

Responding to Shipman

Almost all general practitioners have been distressed that one of their number was quietly murdering his patients while disguised by the shield of professional virtue. Although general practitioners cannot be held responsible for the breach of trust perpetrated by Shipman, they do have responsibility for responding to what happened. The appropriateness of that response may be judged by whether or not it is likely to justify the restoration of patient trust in regulation and monitoring systems. If these systems fail to give patients confidence that incompetent or malicious doctors would be detected quickly and dealt with, general practitioners might then be accused of being unworthy of trust.

A few weeks after the publication of the review in January 2001, I attended a meeting at Dukinfield Town Hall of the relatives and loved ones of Shipman's victims. Around 100 people were present, and because of the conclusions reached in the review about the level of suspicion attached to the deaths, each person was coming to terms with the conclusion that one or more of their relatives had probably been killed by their general practitioner. The purpose of the meeting was for me to explain the findings of the review, and to answer questions about what had happened. The discussion turned to cremation certification. Why had this system failed to raise the alarm? Someone in the room said 'Ash cash, that's what they call it'.

There are points that can be made in defence of the cremation procedures. Ultimately they did cause the alarm to be raised, although not until just six months before Shipman's eventual arrest, by which time he had already killed well over 200 people. The discussion between two doctors of the care given to a deceased patient can be an opportunity for reflection and learning – provided that the doctors are open and truthful. Doctors do generally take care to complete the forms accurately, although there is evidence that this is not always the case.[10] However, these are weak points to make to people who are trying to come to terms with the killing of a relative by their trusted general practitioner.

My response was to agree that the cremation procedures had failed their relatives. As a general practitioner, I had completed cremation forms on many occasions, and it was impossible not to feel some shame at having participated in a patently inadequate system. The response of general practitioners to Shipman's crimes will include a considered judgement of the system failures, but my experience of that meeting at Dukinfield leads me to the conclusion that more is required. The response is also a duty owed by general practitioners to the gentle but betrayed victims of Shipman and their relatives. The response must begin with the acceptance of that duty. I wish all general practitioners could have stood in front of that audience, and breathed in the smell of trust betrayed, and understood and accepted the duty now placed on us.

Work has already started in response to the recommendations listed in Box 3.1. For example, the Home Office[19] has undertaken a review of death certification, and the coroner service is under review.[20] System reform will follow. All health professionals have a role in ensuring that the reforms are workable and increase the likelihood that a future Shipman would be detected. The uncertain patient might also expect the professions to consider what lessons are important for training and continuing professional development, or in relation to revalidation. For example, are doctors sufficiently trained in the completion of death and cremation certificates?

Doctors have another potential role to play. No system is perfect, and from time to time improvement must be introduced based on accumulated experience. It follows that a formal process for appraising the new death certification and monitoring systems could be advantageous. Since doctors will be making daily use of the new systems, they will be best placed to recognise weaknesses and suggest solutions. The creation of a practical mechanism for collating these observations and using them to refine the new system would reduce the risk of future system failure.

Programmes for the reporting and analysis of adverse events in primary care are in preparation, and have already been introduced in hospitals. General practitioners need to take part in such programmes, actively reporting adverse events and promoting action on the lessons learned. For example, the reporting of adverse events or errors with regard to controlled drug prescribing, recording or disposal could lead to a reduced risk of misuse of these drugs by health professionals. The reporting of errors in the completion of death certificates would have a role to play in maintaining these procedures.

The final matter that requires a response from general practitioners is the place of monitoring in the management of general practice. The consequence of the real or apparent decline in trust is the introduction of new controls, regulations and monitoring (*see* Chapter 6). With each new adverse event it seems that new controls are adopted, until the performance of the individual practitioner becomes heavily micro-managed,[14] a situation that is inevitably restricting professional judgement and clinical discretion. Patients are also unlikely to welcome the micro-management of healthcare, since it would be more difficult to take their own preferences and individual circumstances into account.[21] When the pressure for increased accountability is allied to plans to link payment of general practitioners with detailed measurement of performance,[22] control over the general practitioners' clinical decision making could become too restrictive. General practitioners must therefore undertake a comprehensive appraisal of the systems for monitoring and regulating their profession. Those components of accountability that are currently in place and which are not essential should be abandoned. General practitioners need to decide, in concert with patients and managers, the genuinely important outcomes of their work, and focus monitoring and accountability on the latter.[23] A degree of self-governance over the other aspects of care would assist in the restoration of public service and professionalism, and enable care to be tailored to the individual patient.

- The Shipman Inquiry concluded that Harold Shipman definitely killed 215 patients between March 1975 and June 1998.
- The most common victims were women aged 75 years or over, although younger women were killed, as were some men.
- The motive for Shipman's killings is unclear. He was a devious murderer who breached the trust of his patients.
- Various monitoring systems failed to detect Shipman at an early stage (cremation certification, referral of deaths to the coroner, prescribing of controlled drugs), and these will be reformed.
- The medical profession does need to appraise its systems of monitoring and regulation.
- It will not be in the patient's best interest if the current pressure for accountability leads to the micro-management of general practitioners.

References

1   The Shipman Inquiry (Chairman: Dame Janet Smith DBE) (2002) *First Report. Volume One. Death disguised*. The Shipman Inquiry, Manchester; www.the-shipman-inquiry.org.uk

2   Baker R (2001) *Harold Shipman's Clinical Practice, 1974–1998*. The Stationery Office, London; www.doh.gov.uk/hshipmanpractice

3   Smith G (2000) Reporting Shipman. *Hoolet* **winter issue**; www.hoolet.org.uk/28hoolet/shipman/htm

4   Wyndham R (2000) Second opinion: a little perspective on Shipman, true meaning of a free NHS, and the new millennium bug. *BMA News Rev.* **March issue**: 35.

5   Neighbour R (2002) Behind the lines. *Br J Gen Pract.* **52**: 789.

6   Bogle I (2001) Doctors must not be driven out of practice. *BMA News Rev.* **February issue**: 25.

7   Pringle M (2000) The Shipman inquiry: implications for the public's trust in doctors. *Br J Gen Pract.* **50**: 355–6.

8   O'Neill O (2000) Doctor as murderer. Death certification needs tightening up, but still might not have stopped Shipman (editorial). *BMJ.* **320**: 329–30; and O'Neill O (2002) *Called to Account. BBC Reith Lecture 3*; www.bbc.co.uk/radio4/reith2002

9   Horton R (2001) The real lessons from Harold Frederick Shipman (editorial). *Lancet.* **357**: 82–3.

10 Horner JS and Horner JW (1998) Do doctors read forms? A one-year audit of medical certificates submitted to a crematorium. *J R Soc Med.* **91**: 371–6.

11 Greenfield PR (1981) The work of the English Regional Medical Service. *Health Trends.* **13**: 61–3.

12 Moss P, Jankhania J, Upton D and Baker R (2002) *Reducing Leakage of Prescription Drugs*. Department of General Practice & Primary Health Care, University of Leicester.

13 Hall MA, Dugan E, Zheng B and Mishra AK (2001) Trust in physicians and medical institutions: what is it, can it be measured, and does it matter? *Milbank Q.* **79**: 613–39.

14 Mechanic D (1998) The functions and limitations of trust in the provision of medical care. *J Health Politics Policy Law.* **23**: 661–86.

15 Leiden B and Hyman MR (2001) An improved scale for assessing patients' trust in their physician. *Health Market Q.* **19**: 23–42.

16 Mainous AG III, Baker R, Love MM, Gray DP and Gill JM (2001) Continuity of care and trust in one's physician: evidence from primary care in the United States and the United Kingdom. *Fam Med.* **33**: 22–7.

17 Baker R, Mainous AG III, Gray DP and Love MM (2003) Exploration of the relationship between continuity, trust in regular doctors, and patient satisfaction with consultations with family doctors. *Scand J Prim Health Care.* **21**: 27–32.

18 Davies HTO and Rundall TG (2000) Managing patient trust in managed care. *Milbank Q.* **78**: 609–24.

19 Home Office (2001) *Report of the Home Office Review of Death Certification*; www.homeoffice-gov.uk/ccpd/coroners.htm#shipman

20 Review of Coroner Services (2002) *Consultation Document*; www.coroners review.org.uk/docs/Coroner_Report.pdf

21 Hofmann B (2002) Respect for patients' dignity in primary health care: a critical appraisal. *Scand J Prim Health Care.* **20**: 88–91.

22 General Practitioners Committee (2002) *Your Contract, Your Future*. British Medical Association, London.

23 Baker R, Jones D and Goldblatt P (2003) Monitoring mortality rates in general practice after Shipman. *BMJ.* **326**: 274–6.

CHAPTER 4

The Bristol case: the professional team

George Taylor

The story ... is not an account of bad people. Nor is it an account of people who did not care, nor of people who wilfully harmed patients.
(The Bristol Inquiry)

This chapter explores the implications of the Bristol Inquiry into children's heart surgery, and reflects on the failure of the surgical team concerned.

Introduction

The Bristol case has passed into folklore. It has become one episode in a seemingly endless stream identified in the NHS in recent times that appear to point not only to inefficient and ineffective systems, but also to doctors who seem to have poor professional standards. Do we know what really happened? Putting aside the publications in the lay press, a large formal inquiry has taken place and its findings are in the public domain – the Bristol Inquiry.[1]

What then are the facts?

- Bristol Royal Infirmary is a respected tertiary centre.
- It was providing complex paediatric cardiothoracic surgery.
- Working was hampered by a split site.
- The workforce was overworked, having to cover a large geographical area, and it was underfunded.
- It was a new trust with a management structure that identified power but lacked overall leadership.
- There was a history of the professional groups involved not working well together.
- There were repeated examples of poor patient involvement and poor communication.

What then were the overall outcomes of this? Bristol had poor paediatric cardiothoracic surgical results compared with the rest of the UK. On further analysis, it became clear that children died in Bristol who might not have done so if they had been treated elsewhere.

'There but for the grace of God go I' would be a natural response from many who work in the NHS. Was this a predictable outcome of an underfunded and under-resourced NHS? Were surgeons who were taking on challenging cases (that other centres could not or would not treat) doing the best possible under the circumstances? When looked at in detail, each of these excuses is refuted. Although it was under-resourced, Bristol was no worse off than many other parts of the NHS. Challenging cases were taken on, but Bristol's performance was also flawed when dealing with less challenging ones as well. The surgeons were doing their best, but in an inward-looking way. They seemed neither to take up professional developmental opportunities nor to accept guidance from outside.

The following question must be asked. Were these people 'bad' people? Without a doubt they were not, and this was confirmed by the Inquiry Report. They were not a group of 'Harold Shipmans'.

Now that the dust has settled, is it possible to identify the cause of this tragic series of events? To me, the three issues that stand out as reasons for the Bristol tragedy, and which are all interlinked, are outdated views on the role of professionals, leadership and teamworking. All three issues influenced both the way in which the units worked and the introduction of change – or lack of it – in the Bristol departments.

Professionalism and the Bristol case

In the 1950s, the Bristol method of working might have been accepted professional practice. Professionals as a group tended not to question other professionals' practice, or to make overt statements about what might seem to be less than optimal care. The belief was that all professionals had a personal drive to keep up their own standards, and if care appeared less than optimal to an outside observer, there would be understandable reasons, so one did not need to investigate. Doctors were either 'good doctors' or 'very good doctors', and whistleblowing was not the 'right' thing to do!

The Bristol Report tells us that concerns were first voiced in 1986, that one doctor began questioning the results achieved by the unit in 1990, and that bodies external to the trust, such as the Department of Health, knew of the poor outcomes in the 1990s. Sadly, no one did anything.

Similarly patients in the 1950s rarely questioned their doctors' actions. As a group they trusted doctors and assumed that the medical profession would ensure the competence of practitioners. 'Surely doctors will always be up to date, because, well, they are doctors.'

The world has now changed. Patients are better educated, and can access the Internet to obtain knowledge that was not available even a few years ago. They expect to be consulted and to be treated as intelligent human beings. They rightly question more and wish to be involved in decisions that affect themselves and their families. It is also noteworthy that we now live in a culture where 'if someone is to blame, there is a claim'.

Professionals' values have also changed and moved on. By the late 1990s, the then President of the General Medical Council, Sir Donald Irvine, began putting into print what was expected of the modern medical professional. It was no longer possible to collude with colleagues whose standards were being questioned, consciously or unconsciously.

Sir Donald Irvine outlined modern professionalism as having a series of characteristics (*see* Box 4.1).

Box 4.1   The new professionalism[2]

- Clear professional values
- Explicit standards
- Collective as well as personal responsibility for standards of practice
- Local medical regulation based on teams
- Effective systems for dealing with dysfunctional doctors
- Systematic evidence of keeping up to date and of adequate performance

---

This understanding forms a useful template for reviewing the issues at Bristol.

Clear professional values

As the Inquiry revealed, the individuals involved were not bad people. They were professionals who possessed values, but these had become outdated. In failing to evolve into modern professionals, they had become entrenched in practices which proved highly damaging to patients. In the following sections we shall examine such issues.

Explicit standards

Bristol worked on a system of personal rather than explicit standards. For 'they had no one to satisfy but themselves'.[1]

Although professional bodies continue to publish standards for providing good care (some would say too many standards), it is now recognised that production and dissemination alone are not enough.[3] Certain criteria must be met before standards are accepted and implemented by professionals (*see* Box 4.2).

Box 4.2   What is needed before guidelines are implemented?[3]

- Peer pressure
- Feedback
- Marketing
- Financial constraints or rewards
- Organisational systems
- Evidence-based methodologies

Bristol is an example of professionals applying their own personal standards rather than adopting explicit hospital trust or national standards. We are told that the professional and organisational systems designed to protect standards of care were not operative at any of the necessary levels of the local NHS. At trust level the Chief Executive had power, but they did not wish to be involved at the directorate level. There was a lack of leadership. Leadership is vital for an organisation to be effective. Appropriate leadership brings about a series of outcomes (*see* Box 4.3).

Box 4.3   Outcomes of good leadership[4]

* A shared vision for the future
* A supportive organisational culture
* Evolutionary change

There was evidence that both the trust and its departments lacked this. Leadership was distant in the trust. Indeed, it was noted that the individual teams were run as almost independent bodies. Yet we know that a shared purpose and vision is vital for an effective organisation.[5]

We are told that the Bristol Cardiothoracic Unit collected quantities of data, disseminating and discussing such information within the department in a structured and regular way. Sadly, the Unit did not use the data appropriately, being encouraged by an improvement in one year and hoping, it seems, that 'everything must get better, given time'. Berwick rightly states the importance of leadership with regard to figures.[6] The Bristol case seems to be an example par excellence of this. Given the Unit's surgical outcomes, an external observer might have expected that either the Royal College of Surgeons or the 'Supra Regional Services Advisory Group' (SRSAG) would have acted when poor results continued to occur. Although we are told that both organisations knew of the results, 'old-style' professional values together with the belief that the other body was responsible at the end of the day meant that no action was taken.

In response to this case, the Government has proposed the Commission for Healthcare Audit and Inspection. One hopes that people, as well as numbers, are important to it. The case history of Bristol is indeed educational for the NHS. There is a recurring theme of poor outcomes being achieved and discussed, both within and outside the unit, yet NHS leadership at every level was unwilling to take action. The professionals themselves seemed to believe that if they kept on operating, the results were bound to improve. The Royal College of Surgeons believed that intervention was the role of the SRSAG, and the trust believed it to be the duty of the Royal College. The Department of Health held data that revealed the poor outcomes, yet it seems not to have recognised the significance of what it had received.[1]

The Inquiry Report identified the problem of litigation as a confounding factor in Bristol. Indeed, if there is the danger of personal litigation, it is only human for those involved either to keep quiet about problems or to discuss them in a defensive way. The Report was clear that abolition of personal negligence litigation must be a high national priority if a new culture is to come into being. If not, the blame factor will remain, one step removed from the NHS, but alive and well in the law courts. This change would benefit staff and patients, both now and in the longer term.

Collective responsibility for standards of practice

The Bristol case contains a number of examples of very poor teamworking. The report identifies repeated examples of professionals working in isolation. Reasons for this that were identified included split-site working, under-staffing and poor inter-professional relationships. Complex surgery would seem to be an example par excellence of professionals needing to work together and value each others' skills. Medicine and medical training have historically produced a 'macho' doctor with an 'I can cope' personality. As a result, some doctors do not ask for help when they should, and believe that to admit fallibility is to have failed. One of the many dangers of this philosophy is that people 'just muddle through', believing that everything will be all right in the end. Although this philosophy is now changing, there are still examples of education by denigration and bullying in medical training.[7]

A change in attitudes can only be accelerated by a more educational approach to medical training, and by far greater contact between professional groups at all stages of their careers. Experience shows that rigid professional stereotyped views of others are in place after only a few years. It is therefore vital that contact begins at the start of undergraduate training and continues throughout professional lives.

Multi-professional learning is something that seems 'right', yet for which there is little evidence of effectiveness. However, what little evidence we have with regard to multi-professional learning points to improved teamworking as an outcome. Spencer, a professor of medical education, has said that 'it intuitively seems right to influence practitioners of the new century for whom new ways of working together are an inevitability'.[8]

A Centre for the Advancement of Interprofessional Education (CAIPE) survey[9] found that effective inter-professional education:

- works to improve the quality of care
- focuses on the needs of service users and carers
- involves service users and carers
- promotes inter-professional collaboration
- encourages professions to learn with, from and about each other
- enhances practice within professions
- respects the integrity and contributions of each profession
- increases professional satisfaction.

This is perhaps the crux. Just putting professional groups together, whatever the stage of their development, will not help. Learning has to be based within situations where working as a multi-professional team is important for effective patient care. Such situations help young professionals to see (and value) the input of other professional groups into the total care of individual patients or groups.

Regulation based on teams

We know that good relationships between involved professionals empower teams. Rather than putting the onus on individuals, the team may say 'no' if situations or working practices are unacceptable. Through collaborative working, teams can develop sound internal standards to help those whose professional practice – for reasons of health, attitude or whatever – has slipped to unacceptable levels. Such team members can be identified and removed from patient contact. The team will demonstrate strength greater than that of individuals either to resist unacceptable change or to facilitate the development of more positive changes.

The evidence is that teamworking at Bristol was weak, with team members being unsupported and isolated. There are examples in Bristol of professionals avoiding the fact that colleagues' work was substandard. We have heard of the one brave soul who tried to blow the whistle, was listened to repeatedly, but was equally ignored.

The historical pattern of care in the NHS expects teams to put up with poor-quality buildings, inadequate methods and lack of staff, but to continue 'for the good of patients'. In Bristol, they coped with inadequate numbers of paediatric nurses, cardiologists and surgeons. They accepted surgeons operating on both adults and children. They put up with a mixed-age intensive-care unit (ICU) without clear management systems. We now live in an era when patients are rightly intolerant of low standards. If professionals in Bristol had refused to accept the working practices that led to them being spread thinly over large geographical areas, or if they had refused to work on a split site with all of the organisational problems that this caused, the outcomes might have been better. If team members, such as those working on the ICU, had expressed their disquiet about the age range of patients being treated together, and about the lack of paediatric nursing skills on their unit, lives might have been saved. If the lack of clear medical accountability for care had been not only recognised but also addressed, a management crisis might have occurred at Bristol, and teamworking would then have been more effective, more harmonious and safer.

Dealing with dysfunctional doctors

Doctors have traditionally found this to be a difficult area. No one likes to blow the whistle. The Bristol story is a catalogue of damning information about professional practice – details that were known but not acted upon. Professionals are aware of the poor practitioners in their area, and dealing with such colleagues is a nettle to be grasped, for doing nothing is no longer an option.

Evidence of keeping up to date

Technical skills

Keeping up to date is part of the classical definition of a professional. In the past, professionals did not have to provide evidence of such activity – it was just expected. Here the Bristol surgeons fell down badly.

Now it is clearly more difficult to keep up to date when the routine clinical workload is heavy. There are, after all, only so many hours in the day. For whatever reason, the surgeons involved failed to adopt and adapt to new methods and techniques, and they persevered with those about which questions had been asked. They thus exhibited weakness in skill development, and patients missed out as a result. Skill training theory[10] is now well established, and medicine has no excuse for failing to follow its advice (see Box 4.4).

Box 4.4   Developing a skill[10]

- Develop theoretical understanding.
- Confirm this by verbalising.
- Practise component parts of the skill with supervision.
- Receive corrective advice and positive reinforcement from supervisor.
- Develop skill mastery.

Communication skills

Medical folklore is full of anecdotes about surgeons' lack of communication skills. The fact that a group could get away with this in the past is debatable. Today there is no doubt that such a lack is unacceptable. Yet it is only in recent years that communication skills have become an integral part of the undergraduate curriculum. This area needs to be strengthened and reinforced by being an assessed part of all professional examinations. It is known that many complaints in the NHS centre on communication with patients. Bristol was no different, with examples of failings in this area frequently being quoted. The Report is clear that postgraduate education should include basic training for all, and that it should also offer advanced training, with remedial workshops, for those identified as requiring it. The partnership with patients has to mean more openness from professionals. 'Consent must not mean more forms. It means more communication.'[1]

Communication was poor at Bristol – not only between doctors and patients, but also between professionals. This led to mismanagement and poor care.

One of the recommendations of the enquiry was that continuing medical education (CME) should be compulsory for all professional groups. Simplistically this seems right, and with revalidation of professionals it will have to come about. However, we must not lose sight of the fact that this education must be targeted on needs, not just 'wants'. Professionals will have their personal areas of interest, but must also recognise the needs of their trust and of the greater NHS. Education must not just be 'bums on seats', as it has been in the past, but must also produce measurable outcomes.

What we can learn from the Bristol case

What then can we and the wider NHS learn from Bristol? Three issues stand out for consideration, namely the need for leadership, teamworking and modern professionalism.

Leadership

This continues to be a misunderstood concept. It does not mean being bossy, nor does it demand the wartime, high-profile leader. What it does demand is providing an organisation with a vision and an ethos of quality. Good leaders are teachers and guides, and provide the ethical voice. When they are effective, they facilitate change. Without the necessary change, as was seen in Bristol, an organisation increasingly loses its ability to function properly.

Yet change is painful and demands the following:

- the recognition of a need for change
- effective alternatives
- support for those involved during the change
- the facility to develop the skills that are needed both to bring about the change and to fulfil the new roles required once that change has occurred.[11]

Thus proper change depends on clear, effective leadership.

Teamworking

Good teamworking goes hand in hand with effective leadership, and should be its natural product. Successful teamworking requires the following:

- good communication
- all voices being listened to with respect
- the skills of everyone being valued
- adequate time together
- a shared understanding of the short- and long-term aims of the team.

Good teamworking will bring about a supportive environment where blame is *not* the game, but rather a problem stimulates a review to see why it happened, and what needs to be done to stop it happening again. Effective teams may well aspire to be 'learning organisations', a concept that is discussed elsewhere in this book.

Professionalism

Professionals must now embrace the components of Irvine's definition of the new professionalism,[2] for partnership with patients can no longer be characterised as paternalistic, but has to become (in transactional terms) an 'adult–adult' relationship. Health professionals must communicate as equals and allow patients to exercise their rights over their own bodies. They must also be allowed to make decisions that are informed ones.

Conclusion

The Bristol case was an undoubted tragedy. Lessons are there to be learned, and they must be learned. No one can say 'Of course, that does not apply to me'. The Bristol case demands more effective teamworking, clearer leadership and enhanced professional standards that embody, as a norm, the informed involvement of patients in their care and mutual respect. As the Inquiry Report states, there is a need 'to advance ... a patient-centred healthcare service committed to continuous improvement'.

- The Bristol Inquiry found evidence of longstanding poor paediatric cardio-thoracic surgical outcomes.
- These resulted from persistent failures both by individuals and by the whole team.
- There were repeated examples of inadequate patient involvement and poor communication.
- Lessons to be learned include improving leadership and teamwork, and embracing modern understandings of professionalism.
- The risk of litigation remains a negative influence on admitting, and learning from, mistakes.

References

1   The Bristol Inquiry (2001) *Learning from Bristol: the report of the public inquiry into children's heart surgery at the Bristol Royal Infirmary, 1984–1995*. The Stationery Office, London.

2   Irvine D (1999) The performance of doctors: the new professionalism. *Lancet.* **353**: 1174–7.

3   Grimshaw JM and Russell IT (1993) Effect of clinical guidelines on medical practice: a systematic review of rigorous evaluations. *Lancet.* **342**: 1317–22.

4   Shein EH (1972) *Professional Education: some new directions. Innovators to improve practice and clarify professionals' role in society*. McGraw Hill, New York.

5   Senge P (1990) The leader's new role: building learning environments. *Sloan Manag Rev.* **7**: 23.

6   Berwick DM (1998) Crossing the boundary: changing mental models in the service of improvement. *Int J Qual Health Care.* **10**: 435–41.

7   Quine L (2002) Workplace bullying in junior doctors: a questionnaire survey. *BMJ.* **324**: 878–9.

8   Spencer J (2000) Educating the coming generation. In: J Harrison and T van Zwanenberg (eds) *Clinical Governance in Primary Care*. Radcliffe Medical Press, Oxford.

9   Barr H and Waterton S (1996) Summary of a CAIPE survey: interprofessional education in health and social care in the United Kingdom. *J Interprof Care.* **10**: 297–303.

10 Eraut M (2000) Development of knowledge and skills at work. In: F Coffield (ed.) *Differing Visions of a Learning Society*. Policy Press, Bristol.

11 Taylor GB (2002) Clinical governance and the development of a new professionalism in medicine. *Educ Health.* **15**: 65–70.

CHAPTER 5

The Alder Hey case: the institution

Rob Innes

> The truth is that as you handed over your child to doctors and nurses, you did so with complete trust. ... But when you discover what has been done without your knowledge, without your understanding, without your consent, you feel betrayed – so much so that it becomes difficult to trust anybody in authority.[1]
>
> (The Bishop of Liverpool)

> We ... are discovering that, if we explain carefully why we do what we do, then most families are understanding. However, the rebuilding of trust and confidence will take a long time.
>
> (David Hoskins, Chaplain at Harrogate District Hospital)

This chapter describes what happened in the scandal involving the large-scale retention of body parts at Alder Hey Children's Hospital. The case shows how institutional factors severely exacerbated the effects of one doctor's unorthodox practice, and demonstrates what can happen when medical culture and popular expectations get out of step.

Alder Hey is the name by which the Royal Liverpool Children's Hospital NHS Trust is widely known. The hospital was founded in 1914, and is probably the largest children's hospital in North-Western Europe. It has a first-class reputation for saving the lives of sick children, and a history of medical achievement and clinical innovation. It is an international centre of excellence that treats more than 200 000 children a year. It has also been at the centre of one of the most serious scandals to engulf the medical world in recent years.

The scandal concerned the removal, retention and disposal of infant body parts without proper parental consent. This activity was carried out by one rogue doctor, Professor Dick van Velzen, and his associates. Undoubtedly, however, the effect of van Velzen's activity was made much worse by a range of institutional factors, including the relationship of the hospital with Liverpool University, lack of clarity with regard to coroner's procedures, and the way in which the hospital dealt with the affair once it was discovered. More generally, van Velzen's conduct revealed a culture of 'paternalism' within the medical profession in which parental consent was significantly undervalued.

The activity of Professor van Velzen

Van Velzen was appointed Head of the Foetal and Infant Pathology Unit at the University of Liverpool and Honorary Paediatric Pathologist at Alder Hey in 1988. The circumstances of his appointment were controversial. There was widespread concern that the premises and equipment needed for the new Chair were inadequate. The post holder faced the difficult task of establishing a new university research unit as well as providing a clinical histopathology service to Alder Hey. Beyond this, a senior lecturer post promised by the university did not materialise. This fact alone meant that, when van Velzen's conduct began to cause concern, the authorities were reluctant to take disciplinary action against him, as he could readily claim 'under-resourcing'.

As soon as van Velzen was in post, his new unit began to receive fetus and stillborn babies for his examination and report. Within a week of taking up the Chair, van Velzen issued an instruction that there was to be no disposal of human material. The store of material began to grow, to support his research interests. The technical staff soon realised that van Velzen's clinical practice with regard to the removal and retention of organs was unlike anything they had seen before. Until now, pathologists had only retained sections of the relevant organs and returned everything else to the body, except for the heart/lungs or brain in relevant cases. Professor van Velzen removed every organ in every case and retained every organ in every case.

Van Velzen was employed by the university, funded by a charitable foundation, and contracted to deliver six sessions a week to the hospital as well as maintaining a research programme. He soon began playing off workload demands from the university and the hospital against one another, both to justify demands for more technical staff and to explain poor clinical performance standards. The need to retain so much human tissue was explained in terms of the need to build up a bank of human organs that he could call upon in the future, depending on how his research programme developed.

Professor van Velzen remained in post until 1995. During his time at Alder Hey he built up a huge collection of human tissue, which he stored in tubs at his (now infamous) Myrtle Street premises. His period of office was marked by streams of complaints about his clinical service, and by ineffective attempts by the authorities to exert proper control over him. During his final year he actually spent very little time in Liverpool and made no real clinical contribution. He finally resigned, under pressure from the university, at the end of 1995. However, the extent of his misdemeanours was not fully appreciated until the publication of the Redfern Report in 2000 (*see* Box 5.1).

Box 5.1   The Redfern Report[2]

The Redfern Report found Professor van Velzen guilty of the following activities (among others):

- unethical and illegal retention of organs
- falsifying research applications
- falsifying post-mortem reports

- ignoring written consents to limit post-mortem applications
- lying to patients about his post-mortem methods and findings
- delivery of no pathology service/an ineffective service
- failing to keep a proper catalogue or record of the stored organs
- encouraging staff to falsify records and statistics
- failing to maintain proper accounting procedures
- practising deceit upon the university and upon Alder Hey.

The scandal comes to light

On 7 September 1999, Professor Anderson of Great Ormond Street gave evidence to the Bristol Inquiry in which he described the benefits of heart retention for the purposes of teaching and research. He identified heart collections around the country and made particular mention of the excellence of the collection at Alder Hey, which dated from 1948. His evidence brought the issue of organ retention into the public domain.

The revelation of the Alder Hey heart collection generated some local media interest, and on 18 September 1999 the issue of organ retention was reported on the BBC North West Regional News. On 20 September, the Chief Executive of Alder Hey, Ms Hilary Rowland, gave an assurance that the practice of organ retention at Alder Hey had not differed from that at other hospitals. Van Velzen's collection at Myrtle Street was such that this assurance was inaccurate.

Following the broadcast of the news story, many parents telephoned Alder Hey to find out whether their child's heart had been retained. Later in that week, parents began to query whether, if hearts had been retained, other organs had also been kept. Ms Rowland dispatched an officer to visit Myrtle Street to establish the position. He found about 2000 containers holding multiple organs and many pieces and fragments of tissue, taken from around 850 post-mortems.

As the number of queries from parents grew, Ms Rowland decided to write to all of the families whose child had died at Alder Hey and where the post-mortem had been performed at the hospital. They were invited to contact Alder Hey to be told whether their child's organs had been retained. The hospital now began a desperate attempt to catalogue all of the stored organs. In the interim, Ms Rowland issued a press release denying prior knowledge of the store of organs:

> The hospital is devastated to learn that so many organs have been
> retained for research without the knowledge of the hospital, its doctors
> or the parents.

An initial broad description of the retained organs was sent to parents. When they asked for a full list, the hospital delayed for 48 hours 'to allow parents to decide whether they really wanted the information'. Meanwhile the list was prepared. A group of parents called a meeting on 1 November 1999, at which they discussed their difficulties in obtaining information from Alder Hey, telephone calls not being returned, and long delays in securing the return of organs. Parents only received information if they asked for it, and many did not know what to ask for in the first place. They began to describe the attitude of Alder Hey as deliberately obstructive. A support group for parents called 'Parents who Inter Their Young Twice' (PITY II) was set up. The purpose of the group was to represent and support parents, which it did vigorously.[3]

In late November 1999, Alder Hey management offered to meet with PITY II. However, on 3 December, the (new) Coroner for Liverpool suggested that organ retention was unlawful. The Alder Hey situation became national news again. Parents' anxieties and concerns were heightened. The Government responded by announcing that there would be an independent inquiry chaired by Michael Redfern QC.

During 2000, parents continued to complain of delays, missing information, missing post-mortem reports, and discrepancies between post-mortem reports and medical records. The essence of their complaint was that they had been deliberately misled into thinking that they were burying their deceased children intact, when in fact each child had been systematically stripped of his or her organs, the great majority of which had remained stored and unused. Alder Hey's attitude was regarded as defensive and unco-operative. There was a lack of trust. On 23 March 2000, the chair of the NHS trust resigned, following the Stephen White case (*see* Box 5.2).

Box 5.2   The Stephen White case

- Stephen White died in 1992 aged 2 weeks with heart disease.
- In late 1999, Stephen's mother was told that his heart had been retained.
- Later she was told that his heart and other organs had been retained.
- These were subsequently identified as 'lungs and brain'.
- She arranged a second funeral for 17 March 2000.
- On 15 March (two days before the funeral), Ms Rowland told Mrs White that Stephen's organs had been mistakenly destroyed.
- Under-Secretary of State Lord Hunt demanded an immediate report.
- On 23 March 2000, the Chair of the NHS trust resigned.

The Redfern Report[4]

Michael Redfern's Inquiry set itself the task of leaving no stone unturned in the search for the truth of what had happened at Alder Hey. The result is an extremely thorough report over 500 pages long. Redfern's recommendations cover four main areas, each of which will be described briefly below.

Serious incident procedures and record keeping

Redfern found that Alder Hey had failed to make sufficient provision for face-to-face communication of the news of organ retention to parents. They failed to provide suitable advice, counselling and support for affected families. There was a lack of proper management, which led to the drip-feeding of information to parents, and the information that was provided was frequently inaccurate. The result was that each piece of news that was given to parents had the cumulative effect of exacerbating their reaction. Some families faced numerous funerals as a result of organs being returned to them on a piecemeal basis over a period of 12 months or more.

Redfern therefore recommends that trusts develop and put in place *serious incident procedures*. In devising these procedures, the Trust Board should take advice from appropriate experts in bereavement, pathological reactions to bereavement and therapy. Redfern gives specific recommendations on the review and updating of medical and pathology records, including the receipt, use and ultimate disposal of any organ or sample.

Relationships between universities and trusts

Redfern identified the complex relationship between the university and Alder Hey as a key issue. There were surprising disagreements between the two institutions about who was responsible for collections of organs. The two institutions allowed van Velzen to play them off against each other, and the university was reluctant to help Alder Hey once the scandal broke. Witnesses acknowledged that the worst excesses of van Velzen's practice would not have occurred if relationships between the institutions had been better.

The report therefore recommends that 'whatever the underlying contractual position, the relationship between universities and trusts, in respect of individuals and departments with dual clinical and academic functions, shall be one of the utmost good faith in both directions'.[5] The report gives detailed recommendations on what this means in terms of appointing procedures, appraisals and discipline.

The role of the Coroner

Redfern found that clinicians were not sure about the circumstances under which a death must be reported to the Coroner. The difficulties were compounded because the Coroner (a lawyer) wrongly delegated decisions about whether to carry out a coroner's post-mortem to the Coroner's Officer (a policeman). Moreover, the Coroner did not follow up requests for histology with van Velzen to make sure that they were completed. This allowed van Velzen to retain organs illegally from coroner's post-mortems for his research work. Redfern found that some clinicians applied the threat of a (mandatory) coroner's post-mortem to parents in order to persuade them to agree to a (voluntary) hospital post-mortem. Overall, Redfern concluded that slackness and misunderstanding of Coroner's procedures contributed to the delay in identifying van Velzen's abuses.

Therefore the report recommends improvements to the teaching of medical students so that the requirements of the Coroner's Act 1988 are covered. It makes it clear that coroners must not wrongly delegate decisions about post-mortems, nor should they allow the retention of organs unless this is relevant to establishing the cause of death. The report recommends that coroners should establish proper systems to ensure that any organs retained by the pathologist are specified within his or her post-mortem report. Redfern recommends that clinicians make it clear to parents that there is no compulsion for a hospital post-mortem.

Consent

Under the 1961 Human Tissue Act, a clinician was required to ascertain whether, having made reasonable enquiry, he had no reason to believe that any surviving relative objected to the deceased child's body being used for therapeutic purposes, medical education or research. There was abundant evidence at Alder Hey to show that clinicians did not make the requisite enquiries of parents to find out whether they objected. In fact, the report found no evidence of serious engagement of the medical profession as a whole with the provisions of the 1961 Act, either in medical education or in clinical practice. This was not just a matter of 'paternalism' towards patients, although this was part of the problem. 'The bald fact is that on the evidence the medical profession did not properly consider the Human Tissue Act in the first place.'[6]

The report therefore recommends a whole series of provisions for tightening up the Act and making sure that doctors are trained in its provisions, as well as educating the public in the need for organs to be retained for educational and research purposes. At the heart of the report's recommendations in this area is a quite significant philosophical change from the notion of 'consent' (or 'lack of objection') to 'fully informed consent'.

This shifts the responsibility for decision making away from the doctor and on to the parent/next-of-kin. A doctor might, in the past, have assumed that a parent would be too distressed to want to consider these issues. However, the report takes the view that failure to involve the parent in key decisions concerning their child's body will only serve to increase distress in the future. The reality was that, at Alder Hey, clinicians were *not* always acting in the best interests of the next-of-kin. However, even if they had been, a 'paternalistic' attitude (i.e. restricting the freedom and responsibilities of dependants in their supposed best interest) is no longer acceptable.

Beyond Alder Hey

Several major pieces of work and reports have been commissioned in the light of Alder Hey (and in the light of the retention of babies' hearts at Bristol).

- The Royal College of Pathologists has issued guidelines for the retention of tissues and organs at post-mortem examination.[7]
- The Chief Medical Officer (CMO) conducted a census of organs and tissues retained by pathology services in England.[8]
- The CMO held a 'summit meeting' with interested parties on 11 January 2001.[9]
- Professor Sir Brian Follett has made recommendations for the future management of clinicians working for both universities and hospitals.
- The Home Office has established a full-scale review of the Coroners' Service.
- After consulting widely with professional groups, religious and ethnic organisations and patients' groups, the CMO issued advice on the removal, retention and use of human organs from post-mortem examination.[10]
- One of the CMO's key recommendations was the setting up of an Independent Commission both to oversee the proper return of retained organs and tissues to

families who request this, and to address the question of historical and archived collections of body parts. The Secretary of State for Health duly established the 'Retained Organs Commission' (ROC) in April 2001.

- In February 2002, the ROC produced a consultation document[11] considering the following issues:

  - the respectful use and reverent disposal of unclaimed and unidentifiable body tissue
  - a possible regulatory framework to govern collections of human tissue.

- The ROC has also produced a series of information leaflets to help those families who have asked for organs and tissue from a family member to be returned to them.[12]

In his advice, the CMO issued an important set of eight ethical principles to govern the processes relating to retained organs and tissue (*see* Box 5.3). These principles have been carried forward into the ethical basis of the ROC.

Box 5.3   Principles governing retained organs and tissue[13]

- *Respect*: treating the person who has died and their family with dignity and respect.
- *Understanding*: realising that to many parents and families their love and feelings of responsibility for the person who has died are as strong as they were in life.
- *Informed consent*: ensuring that permission is sought and given on the basis that a person is exercising fully informed choice; consent is a process, not a 'one-off' event.
- *Time and space*: recognising that a family member may need time to consider whether to agree to a post-mortem examination and to consider donation of tissue and organs, and will not wish to feel under pressure to agree in the moments after death.
- *Skill and sensitivity*: NHS staff must be sensitive to the needs of the relatives of someone who has died, and sufficient staff skilled in bereavement counselling must be available.
- *Information*: much better information is required, both generally by the public and specifically for relatives who are recently bereaved, about post-mortems and the use of tissue after death. Relatives may also require information about the progress of research involving donated material.
- *Cultural competence*: attitudes to post-mortem examination, burial and the use of organs and tissue after death differ greatly between different religions and cultural groups. Health professionals need to be aware of these factors and to respond to them with sensitivity.
- *A gift relationship*: the emphasis in all current legislation and guidance is on 'taking' and 'retaining'. The balance should be shifted to 'donation', so that tissue or organs are given as a gift to help others, and recognised as deserving of gratitude to those making such donations.

Reflections and implications

It is abundantly clear that the events at Alder Hey have caused a huge amount of public interest and concern, and have resulted in extensive and costly reviews of policy and procedures across a range of public institutions, not limited to the NHS.

Undoubtedly the combination of 'children' and 'body parts' is hugely emotive. Tabloid newspaper headlines such as 'Monster' (*Daily Express*) and 'The Baby Butcher' (*Daily Mirror*) did not help. There was a serious risk that the whole profession of pathology would be unfairly stigmatised. A number of conscientious paediatric pathologists ceased to practise – either giving up work entirely or moving into another area of medicine.[14]

In view of this, it is not surprising that sections of medical opinion have regarded the whole episode with horror – an unholy alliance of politicians, press and pressure groups. Some have suggested that the parents' real grief has been used as a tool to bash the medical profession.[15] It is alleged that the CMO and New Labour have found in this emotional issue a reservoir of popular feeling from which they could draw in order to extend the tentacles of professional regulation. Alder Hey has, it is said, generated a popular and cynical crusade:

> Medical authorities are now queuing up to apologise for practices that have been routinely carried out for decades – without injury to anybody and with substantial benefits to many. Furthermore, they are proposing to replace existing arrangements with a system that is in every respect worse than the status quo. It is likely to cause immediate distress on a vast scale to families suddenly presented with organs of long-deceased relatives. It will cause continuing distress to the immediately bereaved confronted with a detailed interrogation about autopsy. It will do long-term damage to medical research, which will inevitably be deprived of opportunities for research on post-mortem specimens.[16]

Unfortunately, however, the genie is out of the bottle. The public may not have known about the large-scale storage of body parts for education and research, and some people may not have wanted to know – but now we do know.

In fact, the events of Alder Hey show that it is better that we know – because practices that are going on in the shadows will sooner or later go wrong. The deals struck between universities and hospitals, the informal relationships between coroners and hospital pathologists, and the professional vagueness surrounding uncomfortable legislation such as the 1961 Human Tissue Act all provided a context within which the practices of a rogue pathologist could go unchecked.

Alder Hey revealed institutional practices and professional assumptions that were dangerously out of step with the public mood. It was assumed that what people did not know they would not worry about. It was thought that bereaved parents would want to be spared the knowledge of what the hospital and university wanted to do with their children's dead bodies. However, this merely served to build up rage and grief for the future, when the truth had to be revealed.

The removal of organs for teaching and research, at Alder Hey and elsewhere, proceeded under the cloak of 'blind trust'. Parents were encouraged simply to leave the business of a post-mortem to the doctors. However, when blind trust is betrayed, the resulting anger is intense. One of the most poignant events that occurred after the publication of the Redfern Report was the memorial service conducted in November 2001 by the Bishop of Liverpool. In an unprecedented move, it was decided not to invite Alder Hey staff to this service. The destruction of trust was a major theme of the Bishop's address to the congregation, and this was the reason why medical and management staff could not be invited.

The new framework that has emerged from Alder Hey involves establishing 'enlightened trust'. It means ensuring that hospitals keep proper records and so can provide correct information. It means ensuring that hospitals have serious incident procedures that enable them to respond helpfully, sensitively and truthfully when issues arise. It involves establishing a proper basis for trust between universities and hospitals. And it means ensuring that relationships between coroners and hospitals are thoroughly professional. It is a matter of setting up working arrangements, procedures and protocols on which the public can rely.

The key cultural change is a shift away from an attitude of paternalism towards one of partnership. Parents are to be made properly responsible for decisions that affect their deceased children. They are to be given all of the information that they need in order to do this. This means, in part, educating the public about the need for retained organs for teaching and research, in the hope that the decisions taken by parents will take account of the common good.

In his analysis of trust, the sociologist Anthony Giddens describes modern life as necessarily involving a 'risk society'. We are highly dependent on large-scale systems to deliver what we need. These needs include water, money exchange, power, sewage disposal and, arguably, the National Health Service. We live our lives in a 'cocoon' from which we 'bracket out' the risk of anything going wrong with these large-scale systems.[17]

However, life is inherently risky, and from time to time we encounter what Giddens calls 'fateful moments', in which we are confronted with decisions on which our future hangs. The decision whether to marry or whether to divorce, or a medical diagnosis, are examples of such moments. These moments are especially important for determining our identity as individuals. Giddens argues that *empowerment* for decision making in 'fateful moments' is of the essence for creating a sense of self-identity.

The death of an infant is an example of one of our large-scale systems failing, at least in the experience of the parents affected. It generates a particularly intense 'fateful moment'. The way in which the hospital deals with this moment is critical for a parent's developing sense of identity, and for his or her continuing relationship of trust with institutions and indeed with wider society. Giddens' insight is that empowerment is especially important at such a moment. The Alder Hey experience suggests that health professionals need to reflect carefully on this insight.

- The Alder Hey case was not just about Professor van Velzen. More significantly, it highlighted a range of institutional issues which eroded trust.
- An older medical culture of paternalism needs to give way to a new culture of partnership with patients. This is for the sake of both patients and practitioners.
- The move towards sharing responsibility with families is reflected in particular in the key conceptual shift from 'no objection' to 'properly

informed consent' by the parent in the case of removal of organs from a deceased baby or child.

- Blind trust in the medical profession must give way to enlightened/ informed trust.
- Lack of trust in systems and procedures can sometimes lead unfairly to a lack of trust in individual practitioners.

References

1   *Honouring the Memory: a service following the Royal Liverpool Children's Inquiry* Saturday 19 November 2001, conducted by the Right Reverend James Jones, Bishop of Liverpool.

2   Redfern M (2001) *The Royal Liverpool Children's Inquiry Summary and Recommendations.* The Stationery Office, London, pp. 9–10.

3   PITY II maintains an extensive website at http://uk.geocities.com/pity2uk

4   Redfern M (2001) *The Royal Liverpool Children's Hospital Report.* The Stationery Office, London.

5   Redfern, op. cit., p. 15.

6   Redfern, op. cit., p. 3.

7   Royal College of Pathologists (2000) *Guidelines for the Retention of Tissues and Organs at Post-Mortem Examination.* Royal College of Pathologists, London; http://www.rcpath.org

8   Chief Medical Officer (2000) *Report of a Census of Organs and Tissues Retained by Pathology Services in England.* The Stationery Office, London.

9   Proceedings and evidence are available at www.rlcinquiry.org.uk/index.htm

10 Chief Medical Officer (2001) *The Removal, Retention and Use of Human Organs and Tissue from Post-Mortem Examinations.* The Stationery Office, London.

11 NHS Retained Organs Commission (2002) *Retained Organs Commission: a consultation document.* NHS Retained Organs Commission, London; www.nhs. uk/retainedorgans.index.htm

12 Department of Health (2002) *How to Start an Inquiry Regarding Organ and Tissue Retention: options for disposal of retained organs and tissue; tissue blocks and slides; return of organs and tissue direct to families.* NHS Returned Organs Commission, London; www.nhs.uk/retainedorgans/index/htm

13 CMO (2001, 37) op. cit.; NHS ROC (2002, 7) op. cit.

14 See, for example, Evans MJ (2001) Leaving pathology: a personal view. *ACP News.* **Spring issue:** 11–13.

15 Appleton J (2001) *The Rise and Rise of Parents' Groups*; http://www.spiked-online.com/Articles/00000002D1D9.htm

16 Fitzpatrick M (2001) *The High Price of Alder Hey*; http://www.spiked-online.com/Articles/00000002D174.htm

17 Giddens A (1991) *Modernity and Self-Identity: self and society in the late modern age.* Stanford University Press, Stanford, CA, pp. 109–33.

CHAPTER 6

The system responds

Tim van Zwanenberg

All changed, changed utterly.

(Richard Smith)

> This chapter describes how the regulation of healthcare professionals has been transformed in the years following the election of the Labour government in 1997.

Introduction

Healthcare professionals working for the NHS are regulated in part by individual contract, in part through organisational 'governance', and in part by professional self-regulation through their professional bodies. For most staff, the contract is one of employment. The exceptions are general practitioners, dentists, optometrists and community pharmacists, who are mostly independent contractors with the NHS.

Between the inception of the NHS in 1948 and the election of the Labour Government in 1997 there were important developments in the contractual regulation of healthcare professionals by the NHS, and in their professional regulation by their regulatory bodies – the General Medical Council (for doctors) and the United Kingdom Central Council (UKCC) for Nursing and Midwifery. However, the four years following the election of the Labour Government in May 1997 saw an unprecedented acceleration in policy development in both arenas, against the background of high-profile cases of medical malpractice and apparent growing public unease. Furthermore, although professional regulation has remained UK-wide, increasing political devolution has led to the emergence of differences in contractual regulation and organisational governance among the four countries of the UK. The examples given in this chapter are generally drawn from England, which has tended to lead the way at least in terms of policy development.

Regulation before 1997

Taking the example of general practitioners, it is worth recalling that for the 40 years following the start of the NHS the contractual definition of general practitioners' work (contained in the Regulations of the NHS Act) was as follows:

> To render to their patients all necessary and appropriate medical services of the type usually provided by general practitioners.[1]

In other words, general practitioners did what general practitioners did – defining their work and determining their own standards. The first significant change in this area was the new GP contract of 1990 and, as will be seen, the traditional permissive approach has now changed radically. The NHS expectations of all healthcare professionals have become more explicit.

The situation with regard to professional regulation has been much the same. For example, although the General Medical Council was set up as long ago as 1858 to regulate the profession of medicine, it was not until the 1980s that it concerned itself with anything more than professional conduct (i.e. adultery with patients, advertising, association (with charlatans), and so on). The first development of note was the introduction of the health procedures. Doctors whose professional fitness to practise was affected by their ill health could be dealt with through these procedures. During the 1990s a series of other developments followed, as the General Medical Council introduced explicit standards of professional practice, a new curriculum in the medical schools, and changes to the pre-registration year. With regard to fitness to practise, performance was added to conduct and health, with the introduction of the performance procedures through the Medical (Professional Performance) Act 1995.

Similarly, in nursing the UKCC's Professional Registration and Practice (PREP) was introduced in 1995, and formalised for the first time a requirement for continuing professional development. Initially, as part of a process of triennial re-registration, nurses simply had to indicate that they had met the requirements, and it was not until April 2001 that any steps were taken to ensure that they had done so. A sample of PREP profiles has since been audited to ensure compliance.

All changed, changed utterly

Thus by May 1997 there had been incremental development in both contractual and professional regulation of healthcare professionals. However, the incoming Labour Government had a very large parliamentary majority and a mandate to 'modernise' the public services. Furthermore, quality in the NHS in general and the regulation of healthcare professionals in particular were to become major political priorities, as the series of cases of doctors' misdemeanours unfolded. In addition to the cases described in earlier chapters, there were other notable examples, including the following.

1   *The Kent gynaecologist.* In 1998 (the same year as the Bristol case), Rodney Ledward was struck off after being accused of a series of surgical blunders. When giving evidence, nursing colleagues reported that he behaved like God.
2   *The Yorkshire gynaecologist.* In 2000, Richard Neale was struck off when all but one of 37 charges of serious malpractice against him were proven. One of his former patients was reported as saying 'he has left a trail of havoc half-way across the world'.[2]
3   *The Loughborough general practitioner.* In 2001, Philip Green was jailed for abusing young male patients. His criminal behaviour had gone undetected for many years.

All of these cases provoked intense media interest, and each was the subject of an official inquiry. In particular, the General Medical Council's verdicts in the Bristol case famously prompted Richard Smith, the editor of the *British Medical Journal*, to write a leader entitled 'All changed, changed utterly', in which he forecast radical change in the way in which doctors were held to account.[3] And with each case there have been the predicted calls for an end to professional self-regulation in medicine.[4]

Regulation after 1997

At least in part as a response to the cases of malpractice, there has been a plethora of developments in contractual, organisational and professional regulation in the first years of the new Labour administration. The most significant changes are described below.

The new NHS

Not long after being elected, the Government set out its intentions with regard to creating a 'new NHS'.[5] A range of policy initiatives was outlined, which would have an effect on the role, responsibilities, accountability and regulation of health-care professionals. These initiatives included the following:

- the development of a national performance framework for the NHS
- the introduction of clinical governance (backed by a new statutory duty for quality in NHS organisations)
- the development of a programme of new evidence-based National Service Frameworks setting out the patterns and levels of service which should be provided for patients with certain conditions
- the establishment of a new National Institute for Clinical Excellence to promote clinical and cost-effectiveness by producing clinical guidelines and audits for dissemination throughout the NHS
- the establishment of a new Commission for Health Improvement to support and oversee the quality of clinical governance and clinical services
- the development of work with the professions to strengthen the existing systems of professional self-regulation
- the introduction of a new national survey of patient and user experience
- the abolition of GP fundholding
- the formation of primary care groups which were to contribute to health authorities' Health Improvement Programmes, promote the health of the local population, commission health services, monitor performance, develop primary care and integrate primary and community health services more effectively
- the creation of a new 24-hour telephone advice service, *NHS Direct*, staffed by nurses.

A first-class service

A year later the Government elaborated its policy framework for quality in the new NHS, through which standards for the NHS would be set, delivered and

Table 6.1   Setting, delivering and monitoring standards

	Quality mechanism
Clear standards of service	National Institute for Clinical Excellence National Service Frameworks
Dependable local delivery	Professional self-regulation Clinical governance Lifelong learning
Monitored standards	Commission for Health Improvement National Performance Framework National Patient and User Survey

monitored (*see* Table 6.1).[6] This placed professional self-regulation alongside clinical governance and lifelong learning as the methods of local delivery.

Clinical governance was defined as follows:

> a system through which NHS organisations are accountable for continuously improving the quality of their services and safeguarding high standards of care by creating an environment in which excellence in clinical care will flourish.[7]

Clinical governance was a new term encompassing a range of complementary processes, which together would ensure the good quality of care. The processes covered humane care, clinical effectiveness, risk management and professional development.[8]

Lifelong learning had previously been incorporated in the following definition of continuing professional development in the NHS:

> a process of lifelong learning for all individuals and teams which enables professionals to expand and fulfil their potential and which also meets patients' needs and delivers the health and healthcare priorities of the NHS.[9]

For the first time, the needs of patients and NHS priorities were recognised as important. No longer would continuing professional development be seen as the private domain of the professional.

On professional regulation, the Government stated that:

> The organisation of professional self-regulation still owes more to history than to the needs of patients in a modern NHS. The challenge now is for the Government and clinical professionals to work together to modernise the framework so that it is fit for the next century.

Standards of medical practice

In the same year, the General Medical Council issued a new edition of *Good Medical Practice*, which set out explicitly and in clear language the duties and responsibilities of doctors.[10] It made the point that being registered with the General Medical Council gave doctors rights and privileges, but that in return they must fulfil their duties and responsibilities. In particular, doctors were told that they must:

- make the care of their patient their first concern
- treat every patient politely and considerately
- respect patients' dignity and privacy
- listen to patients and respect their views
- give patients information in a form that they can understand
- respect the right of patients to be fully involved in decisions about their care
- keep their professional knowledge and skills up to date
- recognise the limits of their professional competence
- be honest and trustworthy
- respect and protect confidential information
- make sure that their personal beliefs do not prejudice their patients' care
- act quickly to protect patients from risk if they have good reason to believe that they or a colleague may not be fit to practise
- avoid abusing their position as a doctor
- work with colleagues in the ways that best serve patients' interests.

Good Medical Practice provided the foundation for the General Medical Council's subsequent proposals for revalidation.[11]

NHS performance assessment

In 1999, the Government set out the NHS Performance Assessment Framework, and explained how it should be used to assess performance of the NHS in the round (covering quality and efficiency) and to encourage benchmarking between similar NHS organisations.[12] The indicators covered health improvement, fair access, effective delivery of appropriate healthcare, efficiency, patient/carer experience of the NHS, and health outcomes of NHS care.

Dealing with poor clinical performance

In the same year, the Chief Medical Officer put forward his proposals for preventing, recognising and dealing with poor clinical performance of doctors in the NHS in England.[13] He suggested that it had not been clear how the quality assurance activities of the medical bodies (the General Medical Council and the medical Royal Colleges) under the auspices of professional self-regulation related to the similar responsibilities discharged by the NHS. He also pointed out that general practitioners, for example, as independent contractors, could not be suspended by health authorities, even in serious circumstances, and that the only way in which they could be removed from NHS practice was via the NHS Tribunal (unless they had been struck off by their professional body). This was the case regardless of the nature of the problem, be it indecent assault, fraud, a mental health problem or dangerous practice.

The Chief Medical Officer made the following proposals.

- The profession's regulatory activities should meet the required attributes set out by Government on behalf of the public.
- Participation in clinical audit as part of clinical governance should be compulsory for all doctors.
- Annual appraisal should be made comprehensive and compulsory for all doctors working in the NHS.
- The present disciplinary procedures should be replaced.
- Doctors with problems should be referred rapidly for impartial assessment by a new independent Performance Assessment and Support Service (later named the National Clinical Assessment Authority).
- Such referral should result in a range of outcomes, including a period of re-education and training, or referral to the General Medical Council, referral for medical treatment, or referral back to the employer with a report that the problem was serious and intractable. In the latter case the doctor would be dismissed.
- Health authorities should be given a new power to suspend general practitioners.

Incidentally, the Chief Medical Officer noted that professional self-regulation was a privilege.

Modernising medical regulation

In 2000, the Government determined to strengthen the General Medical Council's fitness-to-practise procedures under the banner of modernisation.[14] It claimed that during the preceding months the public had become increasingly concerned about the ability of the General Medical Council to act swiftly and effectively when a doctor's fitness to practise was called into question. It had transpired that the Council had been unable to strike Shipman off immediately upon his conviction.

The Government therefore proposed to widen the Council's powers by introducing a number of changes, including the following:

- the power to impose interim suspension or place interim conditions on a doctor's practice in circumstances which, if the Council was unable to act, would place patients at risk or damage public confidence in the profession
- lengthening the minimum period of erasure from the register from 10 months to 5 years.

At the same time, the Council set out its proposals for the revalidation of all doctors.[11] Revalidation was defined as the demonstration on a regular and periodic basis of a doctor's continuing fitness to practise in his or her chosen field(s). Among the profession, revalidation was regarded as a watershed in the history of professional self-regulation. However, it was, something of a shock to the general public that there had hitherto been no routine mechanism for ensuring that doctors remained up to date.*

---

* One of the curiosities of the 1990 GP contract was the introduction of compulsory retirement at the age of 70 years. At the time there were 19 general practitioners aged 90 years or over still working in the NHS! They would have qualified around 1925, before the invention of penicillin, and their competence would not have been tested since then.

In 2002, the Government set out its policy on the establishment of the Postgraduate Medical Education and Training Board. This new body would act independently of government as the UK 'competent authority' to supervise post-graduate medical education and training. It would issue certificates of completion of training to doctors finishing both general practice and specialist training, and the supporting legislation would enable the establishment for the first time of a General Practitioner Register (to be maintained by the General Medical Council).[15]

Modernising the regulation of the non-medical professions

The Government contended that the new regulatory bodies for nursing, mid-wifery and health visiting and for professions allied to medicine met their mini-mum tests for regulatory bodies, and that a reformed General Medical Council should do likewise.[16,17] As a minimum test, the Government stated that regulatory bodies must:

- be smaller, with much greater patient and public representation
- have faster, more transparent procedures
- develop meaningful accountability both to the public and to the health service.

The new Nursing and Midwifery Council (to replace the UK Central Council) and the new Health Professions Council (to replace the Council for Professions Sup-plementary to Medicine) would therefore have reformed structures and functions which would:

- give them wider powers to deal effectively with individuals who pose un-acceptable risks to patients
- create smaller councils
- streamline the professional registers
- provide 'explicit powers to link registration with evidence of continuing pro-fessional development'.

The NHS plan

This was the plan of NHS reform, with a timetable and targets to accompany the massive injection of extra funding which had been announced by the Chancellor of the Exchequer in March 2000.[18] Among its many proposals, the following would have an impact on the regulation of healthcare professionals.

- A National Clinical Assessment Authority would be established as a Special Health Authority to provide a rapid and objective expert assessment of an individual doctor's performance, recommending to the employer or health authority educational or other approaches.
- A new Medical Education Standards Board (later named the Postgraduate Medical Education and Training Board) would be established to replace the separate bodies overseeing postgraduate medical education in general practice

(the Joint Committee on Postgraduate Training for General Practice) and hospital specialities (the Specialist Training Authority).

- A new UK Council of Health Regulators would be established to include the General Medical Council and the bodies regulating nursing, midwifery, dentistry, opticians and the professions supplementary to medicine (e.g. physiotherapy).
- The Commission for Health Improvement, with the support of the Audit Commission, would inspect every NHS organisation every four years.
- There would be a revised national contract for consultants and general practitioners, with an emphasis on quality and improved outcomes.
- All doctors working in primary care, whether GP principals, non-principals or locums, would be required to be on the list of a health authority and be subject to clinical governance arrangements. These would include annual appraisal and mandatory participation in clinical audit.

The plan also promised increased numbers of healthcare professionals, consultants, general practitioners and nurses. With regard to professional regulation the plan was less specific, but again it emphasised that the regulation of the clinical professions and individual clinicians needed to be tightened. It was also proposed that the General Medical Council should explore the introduction of a civil burden of proof. In the event, the Council has maintained the criminal burden of proof (i.e. beyond reasonable doubt).

To support the NHS plan, the Government also set out new workforce planning arrangements, which it said stemmed from longstanding concerns about the way in which the NHS educated, trained and used its staff.[19] It proposed that in future the emphasis needed to be on the following:

- teamworking across professional and organisational boundaries
- flexible working to make best use of the range of skills and knowledge available
- streamlined workforce planning and development which 'stems from the needs of patients, not of professionals'
- maximising the contribution of all staff to patient care – 'doing away with barriers which say only doctors or nurses can provide particular types of care'
- modernising education and training
- developing new, more flexible careers for staff of 'all professions and none'
- expanding the workforce to meet future needs.

Here again the Government complained of 'a perceived dominance of professional interest groups' in determining the content and delivery of training.

The National Clinical Assessment Authority

The National Clinical Assessment Authority was finally established in 2001.[20] For any doctor referred to it, this body would provide an assessment of clinical performance and recommend a course of action for the doctor and their employing/contracting organisation. Only the most serious cases would be likely to be referred to the General Medical Council.

A number of other important proposals with regard to the regulation of doctors were also laid out. These are summarised below.

- To remain on a health authority Medical List or to be admitted to it in future a general practitioner would have to declare any criminal convictions, bindings over, cautions and 'findings against' by professional, regulatory or licensing bodies. This would include criminal convictions or professional investigations outside the UK.
- For most serious offences (murder or any other crime leading to a sentence of imprisonment of more than six months), exclusion from the Medical List would be mandatory.
- The standards that applied to GP principals regulated through the health authority Medical List would be extended to non-principals (deputies, assistants and locums) through the establishment of Supplementary Lists. Once these lists were in place, no doctor would be allowed to work in general practice unless they were on a health authority list.
- The NHS Tribunal would be abolished, and the existing Tribunal power to suspend or remove a general practitioner would pass to health authorities.
- A position would be secured whereby failure on the part of any doctor to co-operate with a National Clinical Assessment Authority assessment would constitute a breach of their NHS contract.

The document also promised a comprehensive overview of the principles governing appraisal for all NHS doctors, as well as heralding a new system for reporting adverse incidents in the NHS.

The National Patient Safety Agency

In the same year, the Government established yet another new and 'independent' body within the NHS, namely the National Patient Safety Agency.[21] This arose from another report by the Chief Medical Officer, entitled *An Organisation With a Memory*, which had reviewed what was known about the scale and nature of serious failures in NHS care, and examined the extent to which the NHS had the capacity to learn from such failures. It identified two areas where the NHS could learn valuable lessons from experience in other sectors, namely organisational culture and reporting systems.

The new agency was set up in order to:

- collect and analyse information on adverse events from local NHS organisations, NHS staff, patients and carers
- learn lessons and ensure that they were fed back into practice
- where risks were identified, produce solutions to prevent harm, specify national goals and establish means of tracking progress.

The relationship between this new agency and the National Clinical Assessment Authority was spelt out with particular reference to any pattern of poor practitioner performance.

The Commission for Healthcare Audit and Inspection

In 2002, the Government announced plans for a new Commission for Healthcare Audit and Inspection to subsume the existing Commission for Health Improvement, and to incorporate the Audit Commission's value-for-money studies in health. It will also have responsibility for inspecting and licensing private healthcare. The NHS Reform and Health Care Professions Act 2002 expanded the Commission's remit and gave it more teeth. It required the Commission to publish information on performance and a revised star-rating system for the performance of NHS trusts. It also gave the Commission new powers to recommend franchised management, suspension or closure of any service found wanting.

Regulation: new structures and new processes

Within a very short space of time the contractual, professional and organisational regulation of healthcare professionals working in the NHS has thus been revolutionised. For example, general practitioners of the future (see above for the pre-1990 definition of their responsibilities) may now expect the following:

- the need to gain a certificate of completion training from the Postgraduate Medical Education and Training Board
- the need to gain admission to the General Practice Register
- the need to ensure that patients are able to see a general practitioner within 48 hours
- compulsory participation in annual appraisal
- compulsory participation in clinical audit
- compulsory participation in primary care trusts
- changes in the arrangements for continuing professional development
- possible referral to the National Clinical Assessment Authority
- mandatory collaboration, after referral, with National Clinical Assessment Authority assessment procedures
- compulsory registration by GP non-principals on a health authority Supplementary List
- obligatory declaration of previous criminal convictions, and suspension from a Medical List for serious offences
- possible suspension by a health authority
- possible interim suspension by the General Medical Council
- an obligation to report adverse healthcare events
- routine inspection by the Commission for Healthcare Audit and Inspection
- obligatory quinquennial revalidation.

In addition to these regulatory changes, general practitioners were also expected to abide by guidelines produced by the newly established National Institute for Clinical Excellence, and by National Service Frameworks.

In the process, a range of new structures and processes has been established (*see* Table 6.2).

Table 6.2 New structures and processes of regulation

Structures
National Institute for Clinical Excellence
National Clinical Assessment Authority
National Patient Safety Agency
Commission for Healthcare Audit and Inspection
Postgraduate Medical Education and Training Board
UK Council of Health Regulators
Nursing and Midwifery Council
Health Professions Council

Processes
Annual appraisal for all doctors
Assessment of clinical performance (by the National Clinical Assessment Authority)
Reporting of adverse events (to the National Patient Safety Agency)
Professional re-licensure (through revalidation and re-registration)

There have been other changes with less direct effects on healthcare professionals. For example, in the wake of the Alder Hey case, clinical academics must now undergo joint university and NHS appraisal, and a new regime of research governance has been introduced into all NHS organisations. Medical and nursing student projects now require the approval of an Ethical Committee. And yet more changes are anticipated from the Shipman case – in the process of death and cremation certification and in the control of storage and use of dangerous drugs.

An analysis of the system changes

The years since 1997 have seen a remarkable change of gear in the arena of regulation and accountability of healthcare practitioners working in the NHS. This has been associated with a combination of factors, including an incoming government committed to improving quality in public services through investment *and* reform, a Government interested in portraying the recent past under a different administration as a period of failure, a Chief Medical Officer (Sir Liam Donaldson) and a President of the General Medical Council (Sir Donald Irvine) each of whom is in their own way committed to reform, a series of high-profile cases of medical malpractice, and a general public with higher expectations of service and less inclination to abide by previously accepted authority. Arguably the other stakeholders (apart from the general public and the Government), namely the professions, have been on the defensive. Given the circumstances and the individuals in key positions of influence, the changes were probably inevitable, but they may not yield the desired beneficial effects.

In just over a decade the NHS has moved from being an organisation based on high-trust relationships to one in which explicit written standards, which are monitored, have become the norm for both individuals and institutions. Professional re-licensure (revalidation and re-registration) is part of this increased bureaucratic control, which is now also being applied to professional self-regulation. It is one feature of what is in essence a complex system overhaul in the NHS. As in the field of public education, there has been an exponential rise in standard setting and monitoring systems, with the focus of attention coming to bear on audit of systems as a bureaucratic proxy for what actually takes place in the classroom or hospital. These techniques of performance management, imported from the commercial sector, are now being applied to public services, which critically depend on the vocational motivation of professional staff. A wealth of experience with the use of such performance systems now exists, and the almost universal finding is that they tend to distort behaviour in unintended ways.[22]

On the credit side, the changes may encourage reflective professional practice, a more structured approach to continuing professional development, and widespread use of feedback tools (e.g. patient satisfaction questionnaires and professional colleague surveys). They may help to flush out poorly performing practitioners, who either seek help or resign. The public may welcome the openness and transparency, through the greater involvement of lay people in professional regulation.

However, the potential benefits may be outweighed by the potential disadvantages. First, professional practice is by its very nature holistic. It cannot be reduced to a series of evidence-based guidelines which can be audited.[23] What is important is that all aspects of human existence are legitimate concerns of the practitioner provided that they are presented as a problem by the patient. This means that the practitioner is obliged to deal with the complexity of each individual patient. Each person and each context is unique, and this is both the joy and the challenge of professional healthcare practice. Inevitably much professional practice lies in Schon's famous 'swampy lowland' where confusing problems defy technical solutions.[24] Practitioners need to deploy clinical judgement for the benefit of their patients. The danger is that increased regulation may limit them with regard to the inevitable risks that they take in using professional judgement. It may also decrease the professional and personal satisfaction which they derive from using that judgement in the care of their patients – in which case both practitioners and patients would suffer.

Secondly, the increasing focus on audit of systems in the public services (e.g. league-tables) may not bolster confidence. Any number of potential outcomes could conspire to undermine Government, profession or public trust (e.g. recently revalidated doctors being found in breach, or a high proportion of doctors being referred into the General Medical Council's fitness-to-practise procedures). When things go wrong it is very tempting to institute greater bureaucratic control, but the net effect may be to reveal or cause even more problems.

Finally, it is not clear how the various new structures and processes are going to work together. They are purportedly complementary, but arguably they cause confusion and unnecessary duplication. For instance, rather than introducing revalidation as a blanket approach for all doctors, it might have been more effective – and more efficient of resources – to strengthen the General Medical Council's system of exception reporting (i.e. referral of doctors into the newly devised performance procedures), while providing appropriate protection for whistleblowers. Government, public and professional trust in professional self-regulation would certainly be much enhanced if the existing General Medical Council processes were more efficient.

Had this happened, the NHS might have concentrated more on the introduction of appraisal as a formative and developmental process for the majority, and less on the assessment of the small number of poorly performing doctors. Confidence that the regulator would deal effectively with the latter might have circumvented the Government's perceived need to establish the National Clinical Assessment Authority.

- There has been a massive overhaul of the regulatory and accountability arrangements for healthcare professionals since 1997, and more changes are anticipated.
- This was at least in part in response to the recent series of medical scandals.
- Of the three major stakeholders in the process – the Government, the general public and the professions – the professions have been on the defensive.
- Explicit written standards, which are monitored, have become the norm both for individuals and for institutions.
- These techniques of performance management, are now being applied to public services, which traditionally depended on the vocational motivation of professional staff.
- The various new structures and processes are intended to be complementary, but may cause duplication.

References

1   Department of Health (1986) *NHS Act 1977. Regulations.* HMSO, London.
2   Horsnell M and Bird S (2000) Scandal of surgeon who maimed 12. *The Times.* **21 July**: 1.
3   Smith R (1998) All changed, changed utterly. *BMJ.* **316**: 1917–18.
4   Abelson J, Maxwell PH and Maxwell RJ (1997) Do professions have a future? Perhaps, if they are not defensive or complacent. *BMJ.* **315**: 382.
5   Department of Health (1997) *The New NHS: modern, dependable.* The Stationery Office, London.
6   Department of Health (1998) *A First-Class Service: quality in the new NHS.* The Stationery Office, London.
7   Scally G and Donaldson LJ (1998) Clinical governance and the drive for quality improvement in the new NHS in England. *BMJ.* **317**: 61–5.
8   van Zwanenberg T and Harrison J (2000) *Clinical Governance in Primary Care.* Radcliffe Medical Press, Oxford.
9   Department of Health (1998) *A Review of Continuing Professional Development in General Practice.* Department of Health, London.
10 General Medical Council (1998) *Good Medical Practice.* General Medical Council, London.
11 General Medical Council (2000) *Revalidating Doctors: ensuring standards, securing the future.* General Medical Council, London.
12 NHS Executive (1999) *The NHS Performance Assessment Framework* NHS Executive, Leeds.

13 Department of Health (1999) *Supporting Doctors, Protecting Patients.* Department of Health, London.

14 Department of Health (2000) *Modernising Medical Regulation: interim strengthening of the GMC's fitness-to-practise procedures;* available on www.doh.gov.uk

15 Department of Health (2002) *Postgraduate Medical Education and Training. The Postgraduate Medical Education and Training Board. Statement on policy.* Department of Health, London,

16 Department of Health (2001) *Establishing the New Nursing and Midwifery Council.* Department of Health, London.

17 Department of Health (2001) *Establishing the New Health Professions Council.* Department of Health, London.

18 Secretary of State for Health (2000) *The NHS Plan: a plan for investment, a plan for reform.* The Stationery Office, London.

19 Department of Health (2000) *A Health Service for all the Talents: developing the NHS workforce.* Department of Health, London.

20 Department of Health (2001) *Assuring the Quality of Medical Practice: implementing* Supporting Doctors, Protecting Patients. Department of Health, London.

21 Department of Health (2001) *Building a Safer NHS for Patients: implementing* An Organisation With a Memory. Department of Health, London.

22 Clarke A, McKee M, Appleby J and Sheldon T (1993) Efficient purchasing. *BMJ.* **307**: 1436–7.

23 van Zwanenberg T and O'Halloran C (2001) Professional regulation. In: J Harrison, R Innes and T van Zwanenberg (eds) *The New GP: changing roles and the modern NHS.* Radcliffe Medical Press, Oxford.

24 Schon DA (1987) *Educating the Reflective Practitioner: toward a new design for teaching and learning in the professions.* Jossey-Bass Inc., San Francisco, CA.

PART 2

Building trust

Building trust requires a variety of models and strategies, different ways of seeing, and new understandings. Exploring the nature of trust as portrayed in literature, particularly in the plays of Shakespeare, opens up one possibility for renewal. Equally, there is a valid role for journalistic writing, with the press having both a responsibility for and an interest in improving healthcare.

Two chapters investigate the proper place of professionalism and professions. What is professionalism, and should it be taught? How do professions sustain their reputation? It is suggested that we may have moved from a 'status'-based society, where professional reputation was critical, to a 'contract'-based society that focuses on quantitative measures of performance.

Yet new approaches which acknowledge error and share risk offer a fundamentally different way ahead. Learning organisations increase both patient safety and professional job satisfaction. Sharing information and decision making with patients represents a shift in the traditional relationship between patient and professional, with professionals needing to revisit old attitudes and develop new skills.

And the therapeutic environment is also important. Dirty hospitals create suspicion, as do underlying attitudes which undermine trust.

Finally, changes in business organisations during the last two decades are described, where a culture based on control has been overtaken by a new emphasis on trusting human relationships.

CHAPTER 7

Listening to literature

Ruth Etchells

All great poets are by their office democrats ... singers of the joys, the
sorrows, the aspirations common to all humanity.

(Charles Kingsley, *Alton Locke*)

It's a vice to trust all, and equally
a vice to trust none.

(Seneca, *Letters to Lucilius*, 3, 4)

> This chapter explores the nature of trust as it is portrayed in great literature.
> It focuses mainly on Shakespeare's plays, but also includes some striking
> modern works.

Standing back a bit

The focus of this book is for the most part one of immediacy – it is the situation
now, and how it might be developed for good in the immediate and long-term
future, which concerns us. Yet to consider this properly means standing back at
some point and considering the issues in a longer-term perspective. For the nature
of 'trust', when and where it is appropriate (even essential), what destroys it and
above all how it might be nurtured are all issues which have most deeply concerned humankind since records began (and almost certainly before they began,
since – so to speak – Adam was persuaded to eat the apple ...). We could use-
fully turn to history – although there what constitutes a betrayal of trust, and
from what obverse viewpoint that same action is regarded as a brilliant, even
admirable strategy, is often a matter for profound disagreement depending on
many factors (gender, culture and politics, among others).

However, literature also offers us an account of and reflection on the nature and
nurture of trust. Concerned less with the objective record of circumstance, and
more with the struggles, longings, aspirations and griefs of humanity, it explores
how, at the centre of *these* is overwhelmingly the giving and breaking of 'trust'.

Shakespeare *et al.*

This is a huge topic, demanding volumes, so all that can be done here is to identify
some repeated insights. To help to focus them, I propose to use some of Shake-

speare's plays as the most timeless and possibly most profound explorations of trust given, betrayed or honoured, broken for ever or renewed, even against the odds. Moreover, Shakespeare's work helps us with a particular difficulty in the present book, which is that we constantly need to hold together the public and the personal in our discussion on medical trust – the professional and the general, the State and the individual, the moralities of the times and absolute moralities. Since it is at these very intersections that Shakespeare writes, we find that he has something to say to us.

Yet I want to begin with the British public's contemporary choice in literature. For when the BBC held a poll in 1995 to discover the nation's favourite poems, the number-one poem, to most people's surprise after 12 000 votes, was Rudyard Kipling's *If*, which polled twice as many votes as its runner-up. And this was in the context of 99 other poems which were lyrical, yearning, dissonant or downright subversive ...

> Please Mrs Butler
> This boy Derek Drew
> Keeps copying my work, Miss.
> What shall I do?
>
> Go and sit in the hall, dear,
> Go and sit in the sink,
> Take your books on the roof, my lamb,
> Do whatever you think ...
>
> Please Mrs Butler
> This boy Derek Drew
> Keeps calling me rude names, Miss.
> What shall I do?
>
> Lock yourself in the cupboard, dear,
> Run away to sea.
> Do whatever you can, my flower.
> But *don't ask me!*[1]

So splendidly a subversive expression of weary dis-engagement from front-line service is about as remote as one can get from *If*, and certainly expressive of the same weariness that many doctors must feel, at least on occasion. Yet the fact remains that there is something in the *If* poem that resonates with an aspiration in the nation's psyche. What is it?

'If all men count with you, but none too much ...'

A serious reading of the poem reveals an important balance in aspiration. The desired public persona is *less*, not more, heroic and true than the inner person. This is the very opposite of our present culture of 'spin', of attention to public image, of cosmetic self-presentation, either as a profession or as a State, via the media:

> If you can wait and not be tired by waiting,
> Or, being lied about, don't deal in lies,
> Or, being hated, don't give way to hating,
> *And yet don't look too good, nor talk too wise ...*
>
> ... If you can make one heap of all your winnings
> And risk it on one turn of pitch-and-toss,
> And lose, and start again at your beginnings,
> *And never breathe a word about your loss ...*

Allied to this, because it springs from the same root, is a yearning for those who are not improperly influenced – ever – by others, whether they are great or low, friend or enemy:

> If you can talk with crowds and keep your virtue,
> Or walk with Kings – nor lose the common touch,
> If neither foes nor loving friends can hurt you,
> If all men count with you, but none too much ...[2]

'To thine own self be true/One and one is always two'[3]

The common root of all this is, of course, integrity – that is, the quality of holding true to one's ideals, as more important than public favour, private relationship or appeasement of hostility. It is 'integrity' which, by its vote, the British public seems to be demanding as the price of its respect or its 'trust' – not 'presentation', nor 'safeguards', but a quality so inherent that neither safeguards nor presentation are necessary. And that it is ultimately 'integrity' which creates the conditions of trust has been explored constantly in literature and rehearsed frequently in public events and private relationships. Conversely, it is the suspected loss of integrity, of 'staying true', which creates that unease which transforms into distrust. Tom Stoppard's moving play, *Every Good Boy Deserves Favour*, from which the epigraph to this paragraph is drawn, is about precisely this. His heroic Russian dissident, immured in a mental hospital (the State's reaction to his challenge), holds on to his sanity and his personal identity by holding together his own political convictions and certain truths – using 'one and one is always two' as a kind of code for moral conviction.

Shakespeare's major plays always have such a character of integrity, as a kind of benchmark against which the evasions, plotting, half-truths and self-deception of the others may be measured. In *Macbeth*, for instance, the play's whole action centres on the betrayal of trust. With his wife plotting the murder of his king, Duncan (Macbeth's guest for the night), in order to take his crown, Macbeth acknowledges that it is 'trust', sacred trust, which is being destroyed:

> He's here in double trust,
> First, as I am his kinsman and his subject –
> Strong both against the deed; then, as his host,
> Who should against his murderer shut the door,
> Not bear the knife myself.[4]

Yet recognising this, Macbeth is nevertheless persuaded, both by his wife and by his own ambition, to betrayal. By contrast, Banquo, fellow general with Macbeth, responds to Macbeth's carefully oblique invitation to come in with him in seizing power, with a reply which sets integrity above all else:

> Macbeth: If you shall cleave to my consent, when 'tis,
> It shall make honour for you.
> Banquo: So I lose none
> In seeking to augment it, but still keep
> My bosom franchis'd and allegiance clear,
> I shall be counsell'd.[5]

And thus he writes his own death warrant. Kent and Cordelia in *King Lear*, Horatio in *Hamlet*, Brutus in *Julius Caesar*, and Cassio (and indeed Othello himself) in *Othello* are all similarly used as individuals against whose integrity the rest are measured. Indeed, Hamlet's description of his friend Horatio sounds like an Elizabethan version of the poem *If*:

> ... thou hast been
> As one, in suff'ring all, that suffers nothing;
> A man that Fortune's buffets and rewards
> Hast ta'en with equal thanks; and blest are those
> Whose blood and judgement are so well comeddled
> That they are not a pipe for Fortune's finger
> To sound what stop she pleases. Give me that man
> That is not passion's slave, and I will wear him
> In my heart's core, ay, in my heart of heart.[6]

This is a comment about a personal relationship, a friendship – but it is also the comment of a prince about a courtier, a tried and trusted officer. That is, what is true, in this play, of the creating and nurturing of trust in the *personal* sphere is also true in the *public* sphere.

'O, my fortunes/Have corrupted honest men!'[7]

There is a little vignette in *Antony and Cleopatra* that involves such a character. Enobarbus, who through most of the play is a servant of the utmost integrity, near its end betrays his master's trust when he can see that Antony, his master, is creating his own defeat by his reckless self-indulgence, in thrall to Cleopatra. Hearing of his defection, Antony sends his 'chests and treasure' after him, with 'gentle adieus and greetings' (this generosity is too much for Enobarbus, who dies broken-hearted, having been too honest a man to be self-content about his desertion). It is Antony who identifies here the true cause of this loss of trust. His own 'fortunes' have 'corrupted honest men'.

Thus when incompetence, bad fortune or failure are the characteristic of leadership, in these plays – as in much other literature – trust is at risk. In Shakespeare's plays such leadership is held by kings, emperors or generals. Nowadays for us that leadership is held by the State, the Government or its delegated officers, or by leaders of Trade Unions or Professional Associations. Loss of conviction or hope that the leadership knows what it is doing (or cares) can 'corrupt honest men'. Human bumbledom or human sleaze can equally turn away the heart. A very good, sharp account of this appears, appropriately, in a book of verse published to celebrate the Millennium, *Last Words: New Poetry for the New Century*, which includes 'A Ballad for Apothecaries'. This is an account of Nicholas Culpepper, which includes the following description:

> ... As a reckless unlicensed physician,
> He was moved to disseminate
> Cures for the ills of the body
> With cures for the ills of the state.

Those 'ills of state' included the monopoly by the College of Physicians of medical knowledge by restricting discussion of such knowledge to the Latin language. His prefaces to his best-selling *A Physical Directory* (published in 1649, with 14 reprints before 1718) include fierce denunciations of the College as 'a company of proud insulting domineering doctors, whose wits were born above 500 years before themselves':

> 'Scholars are the people's jailors,
> And Latin's their jail,' he roared,
> 'Our fates are in thrall to knowledge;
> Vile men would have knowledge obscured!'. ...
>
> So whenever you stop in a chemist's
> For an aspirin or salve for a sore,
> Give a thought to Nicholas Culpepper
> Who dispensed to the London poor.
>
> For cures for the ills of the body
> Are cures for the ills of the mind;
> And a welfare state is a sick state
> If the dumb are led by the blind.[8]

The analogy with Enobarbus and Antony is fair – for Antony read 'the welfare state' ('And a welfare state is a sick state/If the dumb are led by the blind'). Thus there is loss of trust, and confidence in professional colleagues is withdrawn.

The Antony/Enobarbus loss of trust is a personal matter, yet it symbolises something of world importance. No battles are won or lost because of it, but it signifies the flaw that ensures the loss of a battle which is, in the play, the fight for the rulership of the known world. Similarly, Culpepper's personal struggle against the forces of mystification and protectionism is used by the twentieth-century poet for a reflection on the loss of trust, in our own times, in a leadership which seems to be 'blind' to essentials. That is, poets and dramatists press the case that a breakdown of 'trust' at a national level, although it has national, public consequences, is not only related to the sum of individual experiences, but can also always be challenged by the lonely individual, sometimes with far-reaching con-sequences. Indeed, some literature suggests that only through such challenges can such change be brought about that 'trust' is again possible. (There is a wealth of

Victorian literature about this. In fact, novelists as different as George Eliot and Charles Dickens make it one of their major themes. *Middlemarch* and *Bleak House* are excellent examples.)

The Polonius factor

Sometimes the failure of the leadership (king, Government, advisers or politicians) is perceived as primarily a failure of judgement – it is discerned good or bad judgement which can promote or undermine trust. An interesting example of this is the figure of Polonius in *Hamlet*. Polonius misjudges not only the situation, but also the characters of those involved in it. This leads him to give unquestioning support to a murdering monarch, to misread the seriousness of Hamlet's darkness of spirit, and to use his own daughter as a political decoy. However, he is not in fact a wicked man, but simply a misjudging one, and therefore a man of stupidity and folly. (We might note that the great theologian Dietrich Bonhoeffer categorised 'stupidity' – national or individual – as a moral flaw.) Polonius's misjudgements are partly the result of being more concerned with outer appearance than with inner reality, and nowhere is this clearer than in his famous advice to his son Laertes, who was about to set out in the world. At first glance his 'few precepts' seem to relate closely to that twentieth-century expression of virtue, *If*, but the significant difference is that it is how his son *appears* in men's eyes that matters to him, not what he *is*:

> Give every man thine ear, but few thy voice:
> Costly thy habit as thy purse can buy,
> But not expressed in fancy; rich, not gaudy:
> *For the apparel oft proclaims the man.*[9]

As a result, when he utters, by conclusion, the aphorism which has great truth and force,

> This above all – to thine own self be true,
> And it must follow, as the night the day,
> Thou canst not then be false to any man.

neither Laertes nor we – the audience – can give that truth its full due. *We do not trust men of bad judgement, even when they say true things.*

'Something is rotten in the state of Denmark?' – or is it?

What Hamlet has to deal with, of course, is more than bad judgement on the part of the king. He is dealing with a wholesale climate of corruption, generated from the top. Hence the famous comment, 'Something is rotten in the state of Denmark' (which has passed into proverb) is made by no great leader, but by an ordinary officer (Marcellus) long before any of the facts are known. The same is true of Scotland under Macbeth, where no one trusts anyone. We watch the escalation of such a climate in *King Lear* as the King's daughters grow more confident in their abuse of power.

It is a theme that is reiterated in twentieth-century writing, and not just in our contemporary decade. However, a warning is necessary here. Arthur Miller recently published an essay on his play about the McCarthyism era, *The Crucible*, entitled 'The Crucible in History', in which he speaks of the capacity of a community to fall prey to a total climate of destructive suspicion, in which we invent and believe (although proper thought would quickly reveal them to be fictions) extraordinary malpractices in each other. It is like a virus in the human spirit, he suggests – always there, waiting for the appropriate conditions to emerge in its full trust-destroying hideous blossom. Sometimes, as in *Othello*, the conditions are those of ethnic suspicion fanned by some agent with either deliberately evil intent (as with Iago), or with a perverted sense of justice (as with the Salem judges in *The Crucible*), or with a desire for power or money (as, for instance, in William Golding's terrible novel, *Darkness Visible*). Some would argue that in today's world the media at their worst can similarly be – and sometimes irresponsibly are – agents seeking to destroy trust by promoting suspicion, either for their own political ends or to sell more newspapers (recent handling of paedophiles comes to mind). And often, as in that particular example, the suspicions are unjustified and trust has been destroyed to no purpose. Doctors have been at the receiving end of this as much as any professional group, so the following heart-cry speaks for them:

> *To the Enemy*
> Sit down, have a chair, and relax,
> you who've made former friends bleed.
> Here are all my questionable expenses
> For the taxman, the faithless, to read.
>
> Okay, so I drink, talk to strangers,
> loudly befriending at parties
> those lacking power, position or wealth,
> who aren't distinguished or arty …
>
> Please outline what's wrong with my life-plan,
> help map the route of my passions,
> edit me into comfortable style
> according to science or fashion.
>
> It's not that I don't have ambition
> or a liking for money or fame.
> Is it just that I misinterpret the rules?
> *Don't I cheat enough at the game?*[10]

'He tosses at night who at noon-day found no truth'[11]

Such a climate of suspicion is destructive enough of trust, without any objective cause, and it has always been essential to distinguish it as something requiring a different response from trust lost for good reason (because there has been some genuine betrayal or some major misdemeanour). Sometimes such actual wrongs grow from a climate which encourages them, as the poem above half suggests. (The issues surrounding Alder Hey seem to me to be such a case, where the medical microclimate encouraged actions which the outside world would have found repugnant. Medical 'body-snatching' in earlier centuries grew from the same inner climate, as Iain Pears' rather grisly recreation in his recent novel *An Instance of the Fingerpost* suggests.) So what is at issue here is how far one has become, either professionally or personally, so much a creature of one's cultural climate that personal moral judgement becomes subordinate to it. Rosencrantz and Guilden-stern are very good examples of this in *Hamlet*, betraying friendship to become the corrupt king's puppets, for the sake of what is obliquely referred to as a 'king's remembrance'.

Sometimes, as in that case, it is simply wealth which supplies the dynamic and destroys the trust. Derek Walcott is gloomy in his assessment of the endemic nature of greed in humanity. For him – as for many, reviewing a Western world that is entirely fuelled and valued by market forces – Eden's apple is, so to speak, for sale:

> so when Adam was exiled
> to our New Eden, in the ark's gut
> the coined snake coiled there for good
> fellowship also, that was willed.
>
> Adam had an idea.
> he and the snake would share
> The loss of Eden for a profit . . .
> So both made the New World. And it looked good.'[12]

'Happy, happy perfidy'

Sometimes, however, the pervasive culture is more subtly corrupt than this. I have pointed out that Shakespeare's way is to illuminate the public state by the personal, and it is certainly possible to argue, today as in Elizabethan England, that where there is a culture that accepts personal perfidy (e.g. in personal rela-tionships), there is also engendered a potential for cynicism about public and professional matters. Stephen Spender has caught precisely this moral sequence in his poem 'Song', a couple of verses from which focus the issue:

> Lightly, lightly from my sleep
> She stole, our vows of dew to break,
> Upon a day of melting rain
> Another love to take;
> Her happy, happy perfidy
> Was justified, was justified
> Since compulsive needs of sense,
> Clamour to be satisfied
> And she was never one to miss
> The plausible happiness
> Of a new experience.

> I, who stand beneath a bitter
> Blasted tree, with the green life
> Of summer joy cut from my side
> By that self-justifying knife,
> In my exiled misery
> Were justified, were justified
> If upon two lives I preyed
> Or punished with my suicide,
> Or murdered pity in my heart
> Or two other lives did part
> *To make the world pay what I paid.*[13]

If perfidy – betrayal of trust – is 'OK' in the general climate, then so, he suggests, is revenge, self-murder, the destruction of other people's happiness ... a whole sequence of consequences all arising from the acceptability of personal breaking of trust.

'Close the doors, they're coming through the windows ...'

Sometimes that microclimate is no longer a local cultural or professional matter but has become that of the nation, or of the known world. *King Lear* is a good example of this where, power having been handed over to the ruthless, cruel and self-seeking, the world has become a wilderness typified by a storm-wracked blasted heath, where Lear recognises the failures of power and social organisation:

> Poor naked wretches, whereso'er you are,
> That bide the pelting of this pitiless storm,
> How shall your houseless heads and unfed sides,
> Your looped and window'd raggedness, defend you
> From seasons such as these? O, I have ta'en
> Too little care of this! Take physic, pomp;
> Expose thyself to feel what wretches feel,
> That thou may'st shake the superflux to them,
> And show the heavens more just.[14]

There are times in the history of most peoples, or in the development of most professions, when the whole ambience makes the creation of that tough yet delicate net which is 'trust' overwhelmingly difficult – when the most powerful instinct is to put up the shutters and bar the doors. In contemporary terms, could this mean building up more and more lines of 'security' in the form of targets, assessments and watchdogs? Or professional conditions of service and guarded positions?

'Newsreel'
THRONGS IN THE STREETS
LUNATIC BLOWS UP PITTSBURGH BANK
Krishnamurti Here Says His Message Is
World Happiness

> *Close the doors*
> *They are coming*
> *Through the windows*
> AMERICAN MARINES LAND IN NICARAGUA TO
> PROTECT ALIENS
> PANGALOS CAUGHT; PRISONER IN ATHENS
> *Close the windows*
> *They are coming through the doors*
> Saw Pigwoman The Other Says But Neither Can Identify
> Accused
> FUNDS ACCUMULATE IN NEW YORK
> the desire for profits and more profits kept on increasing and
> the quest for easy money became well-nigh universal. All of
> this meant an attempt to appropriate the belongings of others
> without rendering a corresponding service
> 'Physician' Who Took Prominent Part In Valentino
> Funeral Exposed As Former Convict
> NEVER SAW HIM SAYS MANAGER
> *Close the doors they are coming through the windows*
> *My God they're coming through the floor.*[15]

Drama aside, what John Dos Passos has done here is to catch the sense of a situation that is too large or too dynamic or too complex to control. It is all too much and nothing can really contain it. So it is difficult to trust anyone who says they are trying to put it right – the bank is not secure, the guru's 'world-happiness' is not self-evident, the protecting soldiers are invaders, the witnesses are confused, the 'physician' isn't one, and the manager turns a blind eye …

But! Kent stays faithful, in *King Lear*, the forces of order and good do gather, evil *is* overcome: 'All friends shall taste/The wages of their virtue, and all foes/The cup of their deservings'.[16] Desdemona was innocent and Cassio was vindicated. Macbeth was defeated and the realm was restored. Horatio remained faithful and Denmark was renewed under another, incorruptible and heroic king. In all of this renewal and redemption of trust, is this where, post-twentieth century, we take leave of Shakespeare?

Perhaps surprisingly, the answer is no. There is nothing more terrible in our contemporary literature concerning the breakdown of trust than the scenes of suffering and betrayal in *King Lear*. There is certainly a sense of the apocalyptic – but there is also an insistence that in the face of macro- and microcorruption there is yet faithfulness in the world. There are still men and women who practise the virtues that Lear demanded: 'Expose thyself to feel what wretches feel/… And show the heavens more just'. Mutual reliance does still inform both public structures and personal relationships:

> *This above all is precious and remarkable*
> This above all is precious and remarkable
> How we put ourselves in one another's care,
> How in spite of everything we trust each other.

Fishermen at whatever point they are dipping and lifting
On the dark green swell they partly think of as home
Hear the gale warnings that fly to them like gulls.

The scientists study the weather for love of studying it,
And not specially for love of the fisherman,
And the wireless engineers do the transmission for love of wireless.

But how it adds up is that when the terrible white malice
Of the waves high as cliffs is let loose to seek a victim,
The fishermen are somewhere else and so not drowned.

And why should this chain of miracles be easier to believe
Than that my darling should come to me as naturally
As she trusts a restaurant not to poison her?

They are all simply examples of well-known types of miracle,
The two of them,
That can happen at any time of the day or night.[17]

So what might we learn from all this about how to face and deal with our current crisis of trust? I have described in an earlier chapter how patients need to be seen again as human, by their doctors – and how doctors need to be seen again as human by their patients. The thrust both of the great Shakespearean plays we have glanced at, and of the remarkable John Wain poem above, is that in the full face of sophisticated argument, it is in the end the perception of persons – how they relate and what the profession, the culture and the Government, learns from that, or denies – which must shape professional thinking. Secondly, if our culture encourages perfidy in one kind of relationship, we must not be surprised if there is a spillover into professional relationships. Thirdly, every venal doctor who is in thrall to drug companies or his or her own financial or research satisfaction sets back recovery of trust by another age – which is why it would be so healthy if doctors were encouraged to feel *and speak of* an idealism in their calling, rather than participating in fashionable cynicism. As Robert Frost put it:

But yield who will to their separation,
My object in living is to unite
My avocation and my vocation
As my two eyes make one in sight.
Only when love and need are one,
And the work is play for mortal stakes,
Is the deed ever really done
For Heaven and the future's sakes.[18]

'Greatness without models? Inconceivable'

But there is more. Saul Bellow, deserving Nobel prizewinner for some of the most movingly powerful fictional analyses of our times, reminds us that we do not need to re-invent the moral wheel. Others, too, have faced similar crises. How was the synergy among society restored? Not least, Bellow argues, by looking for great models in the past:

> Oh man, stunned by the rebound of man's powers. And what to do? ... Better accept the inevitability of imitation and then imitate good things. The ancients had this right. Greatness without models? Inconceivable. ... Make it the object of imitation to reach and release the highest qualities. Make peace therefore with intermediacy and representation. But choose higher representations. Otherwise the individual must be the failure he knows himself to be.[19]

'Knows himself to be'

We're back to *If* and the 'self-trust' which that poem demanded:

> If you can trust yourself when all men doubt you,
> But make allowance for their doubting too.

How much of the current anxiety about trust is generated by doctors' own self-doubt? How much have they themselves lost trust in their own profession, and if they have, how far has that rubbed off on a very anxious world? In the midst of unprecedented developments in medical knowledge and possibilities, perhaps the final word that literature has to give to the medical profession on the issue of trust has to do with recovering what has never really been lost — a knowledge of what, at bottom, the whole profession (along with its patients) really wants:

> What is it we want really?
> For what end and how?
> If it is something feasible, obtainable,
> Let us dream it now,
> And pray for a possible land
> Not of sleep walkers, not of angry puppets,
> But where both heart and brain can understand
> The movements of our fellows;
> Where life is a choice of instruments and none
> Is debarred his natural music. ...
> Where the individual, no longer squandered
> In self-assertion, works with the rest, endowed
> With the split-vision of a juggler, and the quick lock of a taxi,
> Where the people are more than a crowd. ...
> Tonight we sleep
> On the banks of the Rubicon — the die is cast;
> There will be time to audit
> The accounts later, there will be sunlight later
> And the equation will come out at last.[20]

- The surprising popularity of Kipling's poem *If* suggests a public mood of longing for integrity and humility over presentation and spin.
- Integrity is the foundation of a trusting relationship. Shakespeare's major plays always have a figure of integrity as a kind of benchmark against which the weaker characters can be measured.
- Literature teaches us that what is true about creating and nurturing trust in the private sphere is also true in the public sphere. So a culture which is accepting of breaches of trust at a personal level will quickly become cynical about trust at a public level.
- Several of Shakespeare's plays explore the adverse impact of poor political leadership on trusting relationships.
- However, we are also warned (for example, by Arthur Miller's recent comment on his play *The Crucible*) against falling prey to a climate of total suspicion.
- Sometimes it appears as if the forces hostile to normal trusting relationships are overwhelming, and we can only act in defensive self-protection (for example, *USA: The Big Money* by John Dos Passos).
- However, several Shakespearean plays bear witness to trust regained. Even in the twenty-first century, there may well be sufficient mutual reliance and faithfulness among us that we can still discover this possibility today. This would need both more deliberate valuing of personal relationships, and a certain idealism among professionals who would be willing to speak and act against the culture of suspicion and cynicism.

References

1   From 'Please Mrs Butler' by Allan Ahlberg, in *The Nation's Favourite Poems* (1996, BBC Worldwide Ltd, London).

2   From 'If' by Rudyard Kipling, in *The Nation's Favourite Poems* (1996, BBC Worldwide Ltd, London), first published in *Rewards and Fairies*.

3   From *Every Good Boy Deserves Favour* by Tom Stoppard, published by Faber, London (1978).

4   William Shakespeare, *Macbeth*, Act I, Scene 7, lines 12–15.

5   op. cit. Act II, Scene 1, lines 24–29.

6   William Shakespeare, *Hamlet*, Act III, Scene 2, lines 63–71.

7   William Shakespeare, *Antony and Cleopatra*, Act IV, Scene 5, lines 16,17.

8   From 'A Ballad for Apothecaries' by Anne Stevenson, in *Last Words*, published by Picador, London (1999).

9   William Shakespeare, *Hamlet*, Act I, Scene 3, lines 68, 70–72, 78–80.

10   'To the Enemy' by Eva Salzman, in *Last Words*, op. cit.

11   From 'Chorus' by WH Auden, in *The Dog Beneath the Skin*, published by Faber, London (1935).

12   From 'New World' by Derek Walcott, in *The Oxford Book of Contemporary Verse, 1945–80*, edited by DJ Enwright and published by Oxford University Press, Oxford (1980).

13   From 'Song' by Stephen Spender, in *An Anthology of Modern Verse*, edited by Elizabeth Jennings and published by Methuen, London (1961).

14   William Shakespeare, *King Lear*, Act III, Scene 4, lines 26–36.

15   From *USA: The Big Money* by John Dos Passos, in *The New Oxford Book of English Prose*, edited by John Gross and published by Oxford University Press, Oxford (1998).

16   *King Lear*, Act V, Scene 3, lines 302–4.

17   'This above all, so precious and remarkable' (first line) by John Wain, in *This Day and Age. An Anthology of Modern Poetry in English*, edited by S Hewitt and published by Edward Arnold, London (1960).

18   'Two Tramps in Mud Time' by Robert Frost, in *The Complete Poems of Robert Frost*, published by Jonathan Cape Ltd, London (1951).

19   From *Mr Sammler's Planet* by Saul Bellow, published by Weidenfield and Nicolson, London (1970).

20   From 'Conclusion' and 'Autumn Journal' by Louis Macneice, in *Collected Poems*, published by Faber, London (1966).

CHAPTER 8

The role of the press

Louella Houldcroft

This chapter explores the role of the press from the point of view of an investigative journalist. Not only is the press governed by its own codes of professional practice, but also it has an interest and creditable record in protecting the public and improving the health service.

Introduction

Just as the NHS has been turned inside out over the past decade, so the role of the press has come under intense scrutiny. After enjoying years of relative freedom, today's journalists are tied by a much stricter code of conduct which governs not just what we are allowed to print, but also how we go about obtaining a story, who we approach and the way in which we do it.

The industry's 'Code of Practice' covers all newspaper, magazine and broadcast journalists, and is written and revised by the Press Complaints Committee, which consists of independent editors of national, regional and local media as well as lay members. Referred to as the 'cornerstone of the system of self-regulation', it is designed to protect the rights of the individual while upholding the public's right to know. It is broken down into 16 points that cover all aspects of journalism, from reporting about and photographing children, to accuracy, privacy and the protection of confidential sources. Almost every one of these guidelines is relevant to the health journalist who is reporting on issues that relate to patients and the NHS.

Protecting the patient from intrusive or unwanted exposure, protecting the reputation of staff in a situation where any misconduct or mistake has yet to be fully investigated, and also protecting the journalist from unfounded criticism and legal action, the rules are there to guide the media while at the same time allowing vital information to be made public.

The public interest

Crucially, a journalist's most important defence is that of public interest. This dictates that if a story is pursued 'in the interest of the public' then it is right that it should be printed. Thus while it is right that guidelines should exist – both to protect the patient and to allow the health professionals to continue doing their job regardless of the events that are unfolding around them – it is also vital that they are not so rigid as to prevent the journalist from doing his or her job.

Perhaps understandably, the NHS is still nervous of the media. Despite whistle-blowing legislation, staff who speak out are still frowned upon by the management, and there is a general fear of being misquoted or portrayed wrongly, made worse by the fact that such sensitive and difficult issues are at stake.

Slowly, however, we are moving forward. Gone are the days when an undercover journalist could simply wander into a hospital and start to interview patients without the management's consent. Press officers now act as a go-between, fielding enquiries and protecting the patients and staff from unwanted media attention. However, such a formal route is unlikely to yield anything other than corporate propaganda, which is why relationships between journalists and the medical profession are vital, both to promote individual success and to expose problems within the NHS that affect us all.

Above all, it is important for those who are unfamiliar with the intricate workings of the media industry to remember one thing – that newspapers do not lie. To do so would be commercial suicide in an age when any lawyer worth his or her salt knows that libel cases pay. Good links between individuals in the health service and the press are undoubtedly the key to balanced reporting and honest accounts. If the journalist is given all of the information then, although the angle of the story will always be based on the most newsworthy point, at least the story will be fair. By being proactive and feeding information to the local press, individual hospitals can massively raise their profile as well as boosting the confidence of the patients who use them.

Health and the press

Health has always been an important issue for the media. A potentially controversial area that impacts on everyone's life – man, woman, adult or child – the successes and failures of the National Health Service and the people working within it are guaranteed to sell papers.

Over the decades there have been numerous 'scandals' that have hogged the front pages. In the early 1960s it was the tragedy of the thalidomide children, revealed by the *Sunday Times*, which prompted widespread distrust of the drug companies and for the first time made patients stop and question the treatment that they were being given. In just five years, from the time when thalidomide was first licensed in 1957 to the time when it was withdrawn in 1962, more than 10 000 babies were born deformed. No doubt the truth about the drug would have come out eventually, but the media fast-tracked this process, giving a voice to the fearful few who were uneasy about the drug, and possibly preventing even more children from being born with the deformity.

It was in the 1980s that the reporting of health issues was launched into the public arena with a vengeance when Edwina Currie threw caution to the wind and controversially announced that all British eggs were infected with *Salmonella*. Economically it was a disaster for the country's egg farmers, but for the media it was a gift. Suddenly questions were being asked about why regular checks had not been carried out to protect the public. How long had the industry and the Ministry of Agriculture, Fisheries and Food known of the risks without informing the customers?

Most importantly, however, it raised questions about how much control people really have with regard to protecting their health, and gradually the 'customers' (or rather the patients in terms of the health service) began to ask questions. Thereafter, the media pushed to expose issues that had for too long been swept under the carpet, hidden behind a facade of elitism and arrogance on behalf of both the medical profession and the Government.

In the mid-1980s, a journalist for the *Sunday Mirror* revealed that the first haemophiliac had become infected with a frightening new virus known as HIV. Claiming that the most likely source was infected blood products imported from the USA and being prescribed by the NHS, she was criticised for 'scare-mongering' by many haematologists. However, her article alerted experts at the public health laboratory, who were furious that they had not been informed of the suspected case, which was the first to be seen in the UK. More importantly, this new information empowered the patients, providing them with answers to some of the questions that they were already beginning to ask. By the time the full scale of the tragedy finally unfolded, a staggering 1250 haemophiliacs had become infected, and the Government found itself being blamed for failing to act on the information that it had been given.

The most recent and perhaps most vivid example of how important the press can be in exposing malpractice is that of BSE and CJD. Without the power of the press and the diligence of a few dedicated reporters it is unlikely that this horrendous abuse of public health would ever have come to light, such was the extent of the cover-up. There is no question that a scandal of this kind also makes a good story. Eye-catching headlines and shock exclusives that will poach readers from rival titles are a key element of the newspaper industry which is, after all, a business and not a public service like the NHS. And no doubt there are times when an emotive headline or biased story causes problems for the individual or individuals at the centre of the argument.

The press and the NHS

However, those who are critical of the press should ask themselves how many of the changes and improvements that have now been introduced in the health service would have come about if it had not been for a free press and the patient's right to question their care. Since the Bristol scandal there has been a whole new approach to the way in which highly specialised services are organised in the NHS. Outrage at the number of cancelled operations during the winter period pushed the Government into providing more intensive-care beds for hospitals across the UK. And the introduction of clinical governance means that the profession is now openly regulated to sift out rogue health professionals, protecting both the patient and the good name of the profession.

In fact, by acting as a kind of independent watchdog, the press has undoubtedly played a role in keeping organisations – or rather the people who run them – in check, the fear of being front-page news being a sufficient deterrent. So while there is a huge difference between the media and the NHS, there are also similarities. Both offer a 'service' to the public, and both have a common goal – to strive for the best possible healthcare for the people of the UK.

With regard to the NHS, the journalist has two roles, namely to celebrate innovation, progress and success, and to expose malpractice, neglect and corruption. In 1988, Sir John Donaldson (later Lord Donaldson), speaking at the

Spycatcher case in the Court of Appeal, said 'the media are the eyes and ears of the general public. They act on behalf of the general public.' His statement was meant in a general sense but is acutely relevant when it comes to reporting on an organisation such as the NHS. As a public body that was set up to provide a service to the people of Britain, it is right that the health service should be held accountable and open to scrutiny. However, fighting through the layers of bureaucracy, even with today's patient-led ethos, is not easy.

Undoubtedly patients are becoming more independent, questioning their care and treatment, probing their doctor for more information and demanding the best possible care. At the same time, the medical profession – which has been widely criticised in recent years for its institutional arrogance and 'old boy's' networks – has made considerable efforts to become more open. However, recent scandals such as those at Bristol Royal Infirmary and Alder Hey have put hospital managers on the defensive, so although they have no choice but to respond to press enquiries, they often do so through gritted teeth.

Ultimately, medicine is still – and always will be – an alien subject to the masses. The complexity of the human body, the speed at which treatment and technology are evolving and the changing patterns of disease leave the general public with no choice but to trust their doctor. And it is this which makes the journalist invaluable – not just to the patient, but also to the profession. With a direct line of communication to the people at the top, the journalist has more hope of cutting through the layers of management and talking heads than does a member of the public.

Acceptance of the press by the authorities is vital, and a good working relationship with the local media in particular can prove invaluable for both sides. Thus while a paper's first responsibility is to its readers (the public and ultimately the patients), this does not simply mean exposing cases where the system is going wrong. Journalists also have a duty to report progress, to keep patients informed about improvements, new technologies and success, and to express in layman's terms some of the more complex aspects of medicine so that the patient has as much information at their fingertips as possible and is able to make informed choices with regard to their own health. Bearing this in mind, the health service need not view the press as the enemy.

Reporting bad news

In the NHS – a service that is led by people, for people, treating conditions over which we ultimately have little control – 'bad news' is inevitable. Until recently, the mystery that has surrounded the medical profession has allowed doctors to practise without question. In hospitals, the consultant was in control, and even the nurses simply followed orders and did as they were told. So while on the one hand the doctor instilled confidence in his patients and staff – a vital quality for someone who literally has your life in his hands – people's absolute conviction and in many cases the consultant's own belief that he was right left no room for mistakes.

The GP enjoyed a different kind of 'protection' from criticism, but one that has proved just as effective. In his role as a trusted practitioner and family friend, the local doctor would have had a great deal of influence over his patients, a fact which has been highlighted all too vividly by the case of Harold Shipman. Today, despite damaging publicity for the profession due to a constant stream of high-profile scandals over the past two decades, people still trust the doctor. What has changed is that the twenty-first-century patient is no longer willing to sit back and simply accept the decisions that are made about their health – a shift in attitude that has been largely driven by the media.

The press is the ideal tool with which to highlight negative issues and force debate or action from those responsible. Thus what starts as a damaging story can, in the long term, drive change in the NHS that improves the health service both for the patient and for the staff. Problems occur when a lack of information results in a story that is unfair or inaccurate. For example, if a doctor is suspended, there is a fine line between withholding all details of the allegation – leaving everything to the imagination – and giving a full account of events that could ultimately prove to be false. Again this is where honesty with the press is vital. Informing the journalist of the background to the case, even off the record, can make the difference between a front-page story and an inside-page brief. Armed with all of the necessary information, the reporter can then make a judgement about the story and decide whether it is in the public's interest to be given the facts.

Reporting 'miracle' cures

In the past, the reporting of scientific breakthroughs and new research was left to the specialist journals, which were read only by an elite few with a specific interest in the material. However, as society started to take more interest in its health, so the demand for information about what was available grew, and now these medical breakthroughs and discoveries form a staple part of the nation's daily news. Initially, the filtering through of information was slow and relied on individuals speaking out about their work, or on a few particularly dedicated journalists who were willing to trawl through each monthly magazine. However, as publications such as the *British Medical Journal*, the *Lancet* and many others became wise to the benefits of publicity, they began to actively promote the work of their contributors.

Now newspapers around the country are bombarded with faxes and press releases about the latest 'breakthrough', and already this is starting to cause problems for both sides. From the researchers' point of view, the reporting of every cough and spit in what is often a very long and drawn-out process before a final conclusion is reached is not necessarily a good thing. Patients start to demand drugs that have not yet been proved to be effective, or for which the side-effects are as yet unknown. And anomalous outcomes, which are bound to occur, can cause widespread panic or confusion among the public if they are reported as fact in a newspaper. The journalist's difficulty is that there is now so much conflicting information that it is difficult to know what to use and what to reject. One day red wine prevents cancer – the next day it triggers the disease. The same is true for coffee, tea, and even too much vitamin C.

The recent controversy over the safety of the MMR jab is a typical example. It is absolutely right that the safety of the jab should be questioned by the media, and that a study such as that of Dr Wakefield should be made public and discussed in the public arena so that the people whom it affects – the parents – can make an informed choice. The confusion has arisen in the three years since that first report, as every week throws up a different study contradicting the last one. With apparently no co-operation between researchers in this field – and each scientist demanding his own column inches in the newspaper – both the media and the patients have lost faith in the experts, and consequently the uptake of the MMR jab has taken a downturn.

What is needed here is better communication between the press and the academics. It is no good refusing to talk to the media and then complaining when the article is incorrect, or is biased towards a particular viewpoint, or has given false hope to readers. Information must continue to be made available so that it can be communicated via the media to the public, but at the same time both sides must take responsibility for portraying that information accurately.

Working with the media

There is no doubt that in recent years people's faith in the health service has dwindled. Patients have witnessed a service close to bursting point as the medical profession becomes a victim of its own success. With the ability to cure a vast range of illnesses and to prolong life where there was once no hope, early predictions by the founder of the NHS, Nye Bevan, that there would be little need for a health service by the twenty-first century could not be further from the truth. Instead, emergency admissions to hospitals are increasing year on year, general practice lists are growing, and long-term care services for the elderly can no longer cope. Thus as the service continues to struggle to keep up to speed, it is not just the patients who are demoralised, but also the very people who are responsible for making the NHS work. However, while health is at the top of the political agenda, real changes can be made if those at the front-line are prepared to speak out.

As the emphasis shifts towards prevention rather than cure, and the responsibility for our health is placed on individuals rather than on the professionals, there is a very real opportunity for the media to educate the nation. Through the media, successes in the NHS can be celebrated and failings can be exposed, driving a change that will ultimately benefit every one of us. Never has the need for the health service and the press to work together been greater.

- The press has its own system of self-regulation, including a Code of Practice drawn up by the Press Complaints Committee.
- The press can claim to have had a profound and beneficial impact in a number of important cases, such as thalidomide, HIV among haemophiliacs, and food safety (BSE in beef and *Salmonella* in eggs).
- With regard to the NHS the press has two roles, namely to celebrate innovation, progress and success, and to expose malpractice, neglect and corruption.
- Healthcare professionals and journalists share a common interest – they both want a good health service – and they should work together.
- The media can educate the public and thereby empower them to take better care of themselves and make better use of the NHS.

CHAPTER 9

Teaching tomorrow's doctors

John Spencer

This chapter explores how today's medical schools are attempting, through their teaching and assessment of aspects of professionalism, to produce doctors with traits and skills that will engender public trust.

Introduction

Trust underpins all professional relationships, perhaps more so in medicine because of the privileged access that doctors have to patients' minds and bodies at a time of great vulnerability, and the intimate nature of the tasks which they are expected to undertake. However, in order to gain and maintain that trust, doctors must fulfil the obligations expected by society. Although guided by codes of practice that have been developed over centuries, the basic tenets of what it might mean to be a professional[1] appear to a great extent to have been taken for granted by the medical profession. It was assumed that most of the 'correct' attributes (e.g. altruism, integrity, humanity and self-awareness) were already innate in the kind of people who were selected for medical school, and that they would pick up the rest from their teachers by a process of 'osmosis'. Indeed this often happened through the powerful process of role modelling, and the medium of the so-called 'hidden curriculum' (i.e. those aspects of learning that 'fall outside the formal curriculum, which are often unarticulated and unexplored',[2] but which may have a major influence on the development of attitudes).

However, student selection has in the past been mainly based on academic achievement in science subject areas. Furthermore, role modelling is by no means always a positive process, and the 'osmotic' transfer of attitudes and values can be unpredictable and inconsistent in its outcomes.[3] Thus, until relatively recently, medical students could graduate from their courses and qualify as doctors with very little formal teaching and learning about becoming professionals. Although there might be isolated courses on medical ethics, law and communication skills, there was virtually no opportunity to reflect upon what, as doctors, they should *be* (as opposed to what they should know or be able to do).[4]

'Professionalism' revisited

During the last decade concepts of professionalism have been revisited, largely as a consequence of the medical profession coming under increasing fire – for failing to regulate itself adequately, for turning a blind eye to unethical or incompetent practice, and for continuing paternalism and poor communication. And all this in an era when what society wants is greater accountability, partnership and respect.

Certain core principles and values concerning the nature of medical professionalism have been published and debated[1,5] Probably the most significant in the UK is the General Medical Council's *Good Medical Practice*, which was first published in 1995. Its central philosophy is that 'Patients must be able to trust doctors with their lives and well-being. To justify that trust, we as a profession have a duty to maintain a good standard of practice and care to show respect for human life.'[6] More recently, following international collaboration, the *Charter on Medical Professionalism* was published simultaneously in two prestigious medical journals on either side of the Atlantic.[7,8] It outlines three fundamental principles to which all medical professionals should aspire (the primacy of patients' welfare, respect for their autonomy, and the promotion of social justice), and a set of responsibilities to which they should be committed (*see* Box 9.1). Its underlying premise is that 'professionalism' is the basis of medicine's contract with society, and that public trust is essential to this contract. The Charter is intended to be applicable in all cultures and systems, and aims to promote 'an action agenda, universal in scope and purpose', including education about professions and professionalism.

Box 9.1   A set of professional responsibilities to which doctors must be committed (from the *Charter on Medical Professionalism*[7,8])

Doctors should have a commitment to:

- professional competence
- patients' confidentiality
- maintaining appropriate relationships with patients
- improving the quality of care
- improving access to care
- just distribution of finite resources
- scientific knowledge
- maintaining trust by managing conflicts of interest
- professional responsibilities.

Teaching about professional practice

Recognising that doctors in training should be prepared for the challenges of future practice, the General Medical Council published guidance for medical schools on change in undergraduate curricula in the early 1990s, entitled *Tomorrow's Doctors*,[9] which was hugely influential. Explicit recommendations were made about ensuring that communication, ethics, medical law and other topics relevant to professionalism became part of the 'core' curriculum, that attention was given to inculcation of 'attitudes of mind and of behaviour that befit a doctor' and the personal and professional development of students, and that all of this, where possible, should be rigorously assessed. A follow-up document, published in 2002, further consolidated this guidance. It states that 'The principles of professional practice set out in *Good Medical Practice* must form the basis of medical education', before going on to describe a set of learning outcomes based on these principles.[10] Similar educational developments have taken place across the globe (e.g. in North America).[11]

Many authors have written about the importance of teaching a correct understanding of professionalism,[4,12,13] the need to develop theory to underpin both practice and research,[3,13] and the challenges of assessing the learning.[14] Key aims for professional development while at medical school have also been defined[4,12] (*see* Box 9.2).

Box 9.2   Key aims of professional development during medical school[4]

- To enable students to understand the origins of professionalism and the proper set of responsibilities of the profession.
- To instil and nurture in students the development of personal qualities, values, attitudes and behaviours that are fundamental to the practice of medicine and healthcare.
- To ensure that students understand the importance and relevance of these concepts, demonstrate these qualities at a basic level in their work, and are willing to continue to develop their professional identity.

Medical schools have responded by developing and consolidating teaching and assessment in areas such as ethics and communication, and by drawing themes together into a coherent curricular strand. Such strands have names such as 'Values in Medicine', 'Personal and Professional Development' and 'Doctoring', and are usually part of the core curriculum. Although there is variation in content, the key elements of these courses usually include ethics, communication, relevant material drawn from other disciplines (e.g. sociology, psychology and anthropology), and aspects of 'how to look after yourself'.

Another educational trend enabling the development of teaching about proper expressions of professionalism has been the move towards more explicit definition of learning outcomes. A learning outcome here means the end-point of a particular learning experience – something that can be defined, and ideally expressed in behavioural terms, so that it can be assessed. Many schools are adopting an outcome-based approach in which all aspects of the curriculum are guided by the intended outcomes. The emphasis is on the product – what kind of doctor will be produced – and this drives the educational process. In theory this provides clarity and accountability, promotes relevance, encourages self-directed learning, and fosters ownership. One outcome-based approach, which was first developed in Scotland and has since been adopted and adapted by a number of UK medical schools, defines outcomes in three broad domains, namely 'The doctor as a professional', 'What the doctor does' and 'How the doctor approaches practice'.[15] More specific outcomes are defined within each domain. For example, 'The doctor as a professional' includes the outcomes 'An understanding of the roles of the doctor' and 'Acceptance of individual responsibility for self-care'. 'How the doctor approaches practice' includes 'Appropriate attitudes, ethical understanding and legal responsibilities'. These can then be defined at an appropriate level down to that of an individual teaching session.

However, a note of caution may be necessary. It has been argued that too much emphasis may be placed on those outcomes that can be defined, possibly at the expense of those which cannot, thereby excluding some of the more important areas of doctoring. Not all that can be counted counts, and not all that counts can be counted! In the words of one author, outcomes should not be omitted simply because of their imprecision or aspirational intent. Outcomes in medical education must be wide in their scope, long in their time line and deep in their relevance to professional development.[16]

The rest of this chapter will describe how we have tackled some of these issues in the undergraduate medical course at Newcastle–Durham Medical School, focusing on teaching about ethics and communication – both themes within the personal and professional development (PPD) strand – and on experience in the community.

Teaching about medical ethics

Dedicated teaching about ethics in undergraduate medical curricula in the UK dates back to the early 1960s, when a special interest group was established in London, known as the London Medical Group. This spawned a network of similar groups in medical schools around the country, including Newcastle. Over the next 25 years such groups were successful in delivering ethics teaching, albeit on an extracurricular and voluntary basis, and played a major role in getting ethics on to the curriculum agenda.

Building on the work of Newcastle Medical Group, and empowered by *Tomorrow's Doctors*,[6] teaching and learning about ethics have been systematically increased in Newcastle's undergraduate course over the past decade, to the point where there is now a coherent ethics curriculum, which is part of the PPD strand. The teaching aims to enable students to develop a coherent personal value system by reflecting on ethical issues that are raised by contemporary practice. However, they should also be equipped to revise this in the light of subsequent experience, thus developing the skill of making ethically coherent clinical decisions, while at the same time acknowledging moral uncertainty and ambiguity. Ethics is often taught alongside communication skills, and tutors are drawn from a wide range of disciplines. In line with the principles of adult learning, the teaching aims to be interactive, enjoyable, integrated and clinically relevant and, most importantly, it is assessed at all stages of the course. The content of the current ethics curriculum (*see* Box 9.3) is in line with the published consensus statement by teachers of medical ethics.[17]

Box 9.3   Contents of the ethics curriculum for undergraduate medical students at Newcastle–Durham Medical School

- Basic principles (e.g. autonomy, beneficence, non-maleficence, justice)
- Professional codes of practice
- Confidentiality and consent (including that in relation to children)

- Truth telling
- Ethical issues in relation to the following:

  - the 'new genetics'
  - reproductive technology
  - the impaired newborn
  - termination of pregnancy
  - research on animals and humans
  - child protection
  - disability
  - pharmaceuticals
  - HIV and AIDS
  - domestic violence
  - transplantation
  - suicide
  - compulsory treatment
  - ageing
  - resource allocation
  - cultural diversity
  - decisions at the end of life

- Whistleblowing
- Medical error and misjudgement
- Aspects of medical law (e.g. the role of the coroner, medical negligence)

Three aspects of this ethics curriculum are pertinent to the issue of trust in the doctor–patient relationship, particularly in the light of recent high-profile cases. These are 'Truth telling', 'Medical error and misjudgement' and 'Ethics of research on humans'.

Truth telling

Second-year students undertake a seminar on 'Truth telling', the aim of which is to enable them to come to a reasoned conclusion about the circumstances in which withholding information may or may not be justified. The seminar links with previous sessions on confidentiality and consent. In a group that is led by a tutor, they first brainstorm the issue of truth telling. Why might it be important in medicine? What reasons do we give for telling or withholding the truth? Are there situations where a 'white lie' is justified? In smaller groups, students then address several case studies (using both video and paper cases), including the following.

- A paediatrician talks with a mother whose newborn baby does not share the family blood group, and whose husband has arranged to discuss the baby's progress at an appointment the following day. The woman acknowledges that her husband is not the baby's father, and wants him to remain in ignorance.[18]
- A father who is reluctant to donate a kidney to his terminally ill daughter because, he admits, he does not have the courage, nor does he wish to see her suffer any more should the transplant fail, asks the doctor to tell the family that his kidney is not compatible with that of his daughter.[19]

- There is uncertainty whether and how to tell a woman with severe dementia being cared for in a residential home, who is asking where her husband is, that in fact he has just died on the way to visit her.
- How should a student who has detected a minor irregularity on an ECG tracing performed on a healthy volunteer respond to their question 'Is everything all right?'

The implications of the cases are discussed in small groups, then shared with the larger group, and finally conclusions are drawn.

Medical error

Medical errors, whether they occur by an act of commission or omission, are common. However, while recognising both the inevitability of error (given the increasingly complex nature of healthcare) and the fact that most mistakes are due to systems failure rather than to individual failure, doctors have difficulty in dealing with error when it occurs. Reasons for this may be found in the culture of medical practice.[20,21] Historically, students are socialised to strive for error-free practice. There is an emphasis on perfection, and mistakes are regarded as unacceptable and therefore judged as failures of character. Furthermore, the nature of 'being responsible' for patients' welfare means that, paradoxically, when something goes wrong it must be the doctor's responsibility – a situation that is fuelled by an increasingly litigious society. It appears difficult for a doctor to say 'sorry' – a basic act of compassion – because this may be construed as an admission of guilt. The emotional impact of error on the doctor is profound, and yet they are typically isolated by their responses.[20] Although systems for the prevention of mistakes, and for the identification of them when they do occur, are necessary, it has been argued that attention should also be given to the role played by medical education in the development of medical thinking about error.[21]

In a session during a final-year surgical rotation, students address the issue of medical error. The aim is to help them to acknowledge their own capacity for making mistakes, to recognise not only the needs of patients and their families but also their *own* needs when they have made an error or misjudgement (or are aware that one has occurred), and to develop strategies to respond to these needs. The session is held in four parts.

1 A video clip from the Channel 4 series *Why Doctors Make Mistakes* is used to highlight key issues related to medical error.
2 A case discussion focuses on patients' needs in situations where doctors make mistakes. A potentially fatal error of prescribing for a 2-year-old child who is recovering from surgery is spotted just in time by the mother and thankfully remedied. What are the mother's needs? How would the students handle the situation?
3 Students are then asked to recall a recent mistake that they may have made, or with which they have been directly involved, and to write a short description of what happened. The discussion is then focused on how the student felt, how the situation was dealt with, and what could be done to prevent such an error occurring again.

4   In the last exercise, students role play a series of vignettes (based on real stories) in which a mistake or misjudgement has been made, and then discuss the issues raised. For example, a paediatric doctor gives a baby the wrong immunisation. In itself this is unlikely to harm the child, but failure to give the correct immunisation obviously potentially reduces the child's overall immunity. The child has left the clinic. What does the baby need? And what courses of action are open to the doctor involved?

Feedback from students about this session has been extremely positive. A frequent comment is that there should be more sessions of this nature in the curriculum across all specialities.

Ethics of research on humans

A lecture in the first year aims to raise awareness of the ethical issues associated with research on humans or animals, as well as the concept of informed consent, and highlights the basic ethical principles which researchers are expected to apply. The key resource for this lecture is the General Medical Council's guidance on the role and responsibilities of doctors involved in research.[22] Some of these issues are revisited in a later lecture on ethics and pharmaceuticals. In the fourth year, students are then expected to put the principles into action when they apply for ethical approval for project work. The process is a fast-track version of that required for any piece of research via Local Research Ethics Committees.

Teaching about communication

The fundamental importance of good communication in medical practice has long been recognised, and the benefits are well documented.[23] A good history is *still* the key to diagnosis in the majority of clinical encounters, even in an era of sophisticated investigative techniques, and teachers rightly continue to exhort their students to 'Listen to the patient – they are telling you the diagnosis', as they have done for generations. Patient satisfaction – an important outcome – is directly linked to the doctor's communication skills, as are many other related outcomes ranging from pain relief after surgery to improved diabetic control or psychological sequelae of cancer. Most complaints against doctors have a significant communication element. Finally, there are direct therapeutic benefits across a wide spectrum of 'talking therapies', from simple listening to in-depth psychoanalysis. Nonetheless, as with ethics, *formal* teaching about communication in undergraduate medical education was until relatively recently a minority activity. It usually consisted of stand-alone courses, which despite innovative use of video, role play and simulated patients were largely ineffective. Such teaching was often not integrated with the rest of the curriculum and, most importantly, students' skills were not assessed.

Reasons for this include the prevalence of several myths about communication skills. For example, it is commonly believed that they are:

- innate and cannot be learned
- an aspect of personality and therefore fixed

- best picked up by experience (i.e they are 'caught' rather than taught)
- no more than common sense, and therefore do not need to be taught.

All of these beliefs can be robustly challenged.

However, there has been a major expansion in communication skills teaching (CST) in undergraduate courses over the past decade, influenced by policy documents including *Tomorrow's Doctors*, the Kennedy Report[24] and international consensus statements, the most recent of which was published in 1999.[25]

There is a rich literature on communication skills teaching, and several frameworks have been described to guide teaching, practice and research. One of these is the Calgary–Cambridge Guide,[23] shown in Box 9.4.

Box 9.4   A framework for communication skills teaching based on the Calgary–Cambridge Guide[23]

Initiating the interview
Establishing initial rapport
Identifying the reason(s) for the consultation

Gathering information
Exploration of the problem(s)
Understanding the patient's perspective
Providing structure for the consultation

Building the relationship
Developing rapport
Involving the patient

Explanation and planning
Providing the correct amount and type of information
Aiding accurate recall and understanding
Achieving a shared understanding – incorporating the patient's perspective
Planning – shared decision making

Closing the session

Using this framework, the process of communication can be broken down into smaller units, and component 'microskills' can be taught at an appropriate level.

The Calgary–Cambridge framework helps to promote a patient-centred approach. For example, it highlights the need for the student or doctor not only to gather information about the patient's symptoms and signs in order to inform a biomedical diagnosis (i.e. the 'doctor's agenda'), but also to find out how the problem has affected a particular patient in terms of their thoughts and feelings (i.e. the patient's agenda). Similarly, a major goal is to achieve a shared understanding and involve the patient in decision making. The framework is the basis of Newcastle–Durham Medical School's communication curriculum, which runs as a 'vertical' theme throughout the five years of the undergraduate course. As with ethics teaching, it is integrated with the rest of the course and is fully assessed.

Three areas of communication are closely related to the issue of trust in the doctor–patient relationship, namely 'Eliciting the patient's ideas, concerns and expectations', 'Demonstrating empathy' and 'Involving the patient in decision making.'

Ideas, concerns and expectations

The importance of eliciting the patient's ideas, concerns and expectations (ICE) is emphasised from the start in CST at Newcastle–Durham Medical School. Students are taught that no medical history is complete without this information. Furthermore, it is often the key to a better outcome. For example, a recent review showed that the main factor influencing patients' decisions to follow the advice offered or to take the medicines prescribed by their doctors was whether or not their beliefs about medicine taking were elicited.[26]

The skills of eliciting patients' ICE are rehearsed and discussed in sessions using role play with simulated patients, which start in the second year. For example, during the Chronic Illness and Rehabilitation rotation in the third year, all students undertake such a role play. A typical scenario involves a middle-aged man who comes to see his general practitioner to discuss rehabilitation a few weeks after being admitted to hospital with his first heart attack. Unsurprisingly, he has a number of concerns. He feels as if he is 'on the scrap heap', and he is frightened about the future. He wonders when and whether he will be able to return to work, and he has a 'hidden' concern about when it will be safe to resume sexual relationships. The student is instructed to find out why the patient has come, and to attempt to address some of the problems. The (trained) role player is briefed to respond as naturally as possible to students' questioning. If they use a mechanistic style, with mostly closed questions, the 'patient' will offer less information, especially of a sensitive nature, than they would do in response to a more open approach. The session is videotaped, which allows feedback to be given to the student, including feedback from the 'patient', who may stay 'in role' and bring to life what it feels like to be a patient in such circumstances. The fact that a student's ability to elicit ICE sensitively is rewarded in clinical assessments reinforces the learning.

Empathy

Empathy has been described as 'the ability to understand the patient's situation, perspective and feelings, and to communicate that understanding to the patient'.[27] Empathy enhances the doctor–patient relationship, increases both patient *and* doctor satisfaction with care and diagnostic accuracy, and ultimately improves the quality of care. Current thinking is that empathy consists of a set of competencies that are not necessarily innate, but which can be learned.

Few would disagree that empathy is a key attribute in doctoring, and medical students recognise its importance. However, it seems that something happens during their training which dents or damages their ability to be empathic. In the words of one author on the subject, 'Students begin their medical education with a cargo of empathy, but we teach them to see themselves as experts. To fix what is damaged and to "rule out" disease in their field. ... We first teach them science, and then we teach them detachment'.[28]

The concept of empathy is introduced to first-year medical students, building on teaching and learning about basic micro-skills. A 'scene-setting' lecture outlines what is meant by 'empathy' and how it differs from sympathy, along with evidence about the importance of empathy in the clinical encounter. A model of empathy is presented and practical advice is given about empathic responses. In small groups that are led by a tutor, students then explore the concept further. They are shown video clips of a simulated patient making a series of statements, and they are asked to address a range of issues. The scenario is that the patient, a woman in her early forties, has been diagnosed with advanced cancer and has been given a very guarded prognosis. Her emotionally charged statements include the following: 'But my son ... he's only 12' and 'I knew there was something wrong when I saw the doctor six months ago – of course *he* said everything was alright'. In relation to each of these statements, students are asked to write down the words they would use in response under the four headings shown in Box 9.5.

Box 9.5   Questions for exercise on empathy

- What would you like to say, if the consequence did not matter (i.e. what would be your gut reaction)?
- What would be a platitude?
- What do you think are the emotion(s) behind the statement?
- What would be an appropriate empathic response?

Discussion and debate then follow. Key issues include the fact that gut reactions are common, and may be negative (e.g. 'I don't want to know about this' or 'Pull yourself together'), but this is natural and 'OK', provided that they are not acted upon. However, it is important to acknowledge them and to recognise their origins. For example, the process of 'transference', whereby the patient projects thoughts and feelings on to the doctor which derive from other relationships in their life, is a well-recognised phenomenon, as is the opposite process, so-called 'counter-transference'. These processes are often unconscious, but they can be very powerful, and can inhibit communication and interfere with the development of an effective doctor–patient relationship.

Platitudes are all too common and often unhelpful, but may nonetheless have a place. A platitude may sometimes be all that can be said at a particular moment – indeed it may be all that the patient wants to hear. *How* such a response is made may be more important than what is actually said. This promotes a discussion about the importance of non-verbal communication and the role of touch.

Students identify a variety of feelings and emotions which they think the patient is experiencing, indicating the range and variation in interpretation, and the complexity of emotional reactions (as well as the potential hazards of making assumptions about how another person is feeling and what they are thinking). Discussion helps to promote self-awareness through reflection – a crucial dimension of professional development.[29] Finally, the articulation of empathic responses gives students the opportunity to explore different ways of demonstrating their understanding of a patient's situation.

Involving patients

Much has been written about the need to recognise patients' own expertise, and to involve them as partners in decisions about their own healthcare.[30,31] This recognises patients' autonomy and enhances health outcomes. However, the profession is only just beginning to understand the complexities, let alone teach about them. Nonetheless, competencies and models for the practice of informed, shared decision making have been developed which will guide teaching and learning.[31] A patient-centred approach in CST[23] is a sound basis for implementing such models.

Actively involving patients in teaching is also likely to help to promote empathy and understanding, and in return to build trust. Traditionally, patients have played a largely passive role in medical education, simply acting as 'interesting teaching material'. However, there is evidence that more active involvement may have significant benefits for patients, as well as important educational gains. Students are motivated through relevance and learning in context. The acquisition and refinement of skills and attitudes, as well as the development of professionalism, are also enhanced.[32] However, such involvement requires an appropriate ethical framework, including guidelines on consent and confidentiality which, it is argued, will protect both patients and students.[33] Whatever abuses of patients may have occurred in the past in the 'service' of education, medical schools now recognise the primacy of patient welfare, and the need for both ethical practice and effective risk management. For example, at Newcastle–Durham Medical School all students are expected to sign a 'Learning Agreement' annually. This outlines the expectations and obligations of students and the Medical School under the headings 'Conduct', 'Learning', 'Confidentiality', 'Immunisation', 'Indemnity' and 'Data Protection'. Students are also expected to have police clearance from the Criminal Records Bureau. The fact that serious breach of the agreement constitutes good cause for termination of studies emphasises the importance of professionalism in doctoring.

Teaching about people and communities

Medical schools have been criticised for being remote from the communities that they serve, and have been exhorted to review their 'mission' in order to ensure that the education which they provide promotes social responsibilityand is more relevant to societal needs, as opposed to serving the needs of the profession.[34] Thus recommendations for change have included a higher profile for social and behavioural science,[35] earlier patient contact, and more placements in general practice and the community.[9] There are many areas in which learning in (and about) the community can complement hospital experience or even supplant it. Specific aspects that can only really be taught through a community perspective include the patient's day-to-day experience of ill health and disability, the social and environmental determinants of health and disease, and community needs.[36]

As an example, first-year students at Newcastle–Durham Medical School have a placement with a pregnant mother early on in their first term. The aim of the

'Family Study' is to learn about the impact of a new baby on a family. Students follow the course of the pregnancy and the arrival of the new baby through regular contact with the family, linked small-group work and independent study. They write a project report at the end, which contributes to their overall grades. Having to write a letter of introduction, seek the patient's consent for access to medical records and write the report for possible scrutiny by the patient encourages students to value the patient's autonomy and respect confidentiality. Similar issues pertain with a project in their second year, when students are attached to a person in the community with a long-term health problem. Durham students' experience is complemented by a placement with a community agency in either the statutory or voluntary sector (including local church organisations, youth projects, self-help groups and the police), which bridges the first and second year. Again students write up their experience, looking in particular at user perspectives, their inter-actions with professionals, inter-agency working and policies in practice. Early evaluations of this innovation are very encouraging.[37]

The challenges of teaching professionalism
The learning environment

The learning environment is one of the most powerful influences on motivation. The term 'learning environment' describes the overall educational context, and goes beyond the physical environment to include the emotional and intellectual climates. It is one of the routes by which professional socialisation takes place, and by which values and behaviours are shaped through the 'hidden curriculum'.[2] An environment that is conducive to learning is supportive and safe, fosters collaboration, values the contribution of individuals and is based on mutual respect.[38] Medical schools in the past have been likened to abusive family systems, with characteristic features of 'unrealistic expectations, denial, indirect communication patterns, rigidity and isolation'.[39] Although this analysis may seem unduly harsh, particularly in view of the major reforms of the past decade, it provides an insight into factors that may still be an obstacle to providing an appropriate climate.

Barriers within the institution

A number of potential barriers to implementing teaching about professionalism have been described. Objections include a lack of curricular time, and the beliefs that professionalism is not teachable, that it is a luxury and of less importance than basic or clinical science, or that 'some things may be better left unsaid'.[13] As with CST, there are robust arguments to challenge all of these beliefs.

A more pressing problem in the contemporary medical school environment – in which research is increasingly valued above teaching, with the added pressures of increasing student intake and problems with recruitment and retention of clinical academic staff – is that those approaches to teaching and learning which are most appropriate for teaching professionalism, such as small-group teaching and the use of simulated patients, are expensive and human resource-intensive.

Assessing professional behaviour and competence

It is impossible to overstate the importance of assessment in the educational process. It is one of the most important influences on learning – not only on *what* is learned but on *how* it is learned. Thus it is important to ensure that assessment drives learning appropriately by being aligned with intended outcomes. Ideally an assessment instrument should measure exactly what we want to measure (validity) and, since we can only ever *sample* a person's behaviour, produce generalisable results (reliability). Reliability is especially important in 'high-stakes' situations, such as qualification or certification.[39] Unfortunately, a number of issues bedevil the assessment of professionalism. By its very nature, professional development is more of a process than an end-point. Furthermore, it is a complex construct,[3,14] only certain elements of which may be amenable to assessment (e.g. communication). The gap between competence (what a person does under examination conditions) and performance (what they do in everyday practice) is also well recognised.[39] Assessing behaviour in abstraction from the real world is problematic, given that behaviour is heavily context-dependent.[3] Many methods that lend themselves to the more formative, ongoing approach that assessment of professional development requires, such as portfolios, have yet to be shown to be sufficiently reliable for 'high-stakes' decisions about progress. Finally, although as a general rule the assessment of professional competence should involve multiple observations of specific behaviour on multiple occasions by multiple judges in order to achieve maximum reliability, there are obvious resource implications. In recognition of these problems, much research and development is currently being focused on this area.[14]

Evidence of effectiveness

Evidence of the effectiveness of teaching about professionalism is patchy. CST has the strongest evidence base, supporting experiential approaches that are sustained throughout the course.[29] Evidence is also accumulating that community-based education promotes more holistic attitudes in students.[36] From an educational perspective, approaches to teaching about professionalism tend to conform to principles of student-centredness and reflective practice,[37] and should thus promote more effective learning. However, without a firmer theoretical base[3] and robust assessment tools, questions about the effectiveness of approaches to teaching and learning will not be easily answered.

Future trends

Professionalism is now firmly on the medical school agenda. For example, in a recent survey of 116 medical schools in the USA, 90% said that they offered some training in professionalism.[4] Much progress has also been made in implementing such teaching in the UK.[40] Professionalism has been a major theme at national and international medical education conferences for a number of years (e.g. the majority of UK medical and dental schools were represented at a national conference in late

2001), and it is the focus of many editorials, articles and books, complementing guidelines and charters produced by professional bodies.

Several trends in contemporary healthcare education may enable further development of teaching and learning about professionalism, and may profoundly influence the culture of medicine.[10,11]

- *Inter-professional learning.* Shared learning between health professionals from undergraduate level onwards is one of the major educational trends of the moment. It is claimed that this will lead to better collaboration and teamwork, ultimately for the benefit of patients. Although the 'jury is still out' as to whether or not these aims are achieved, such an approach certainly has a powerful intuitive appeal.
- *Humanities in medical education.* A strong argument has been made for providing medical students with more opportunities to study humanities (in the broadest sense), to help them to develop 'a more compassionate understanding of the individual in society, to inspire empathy with patients and colleagues, and to become more "rounded" people themselves'.[41] In fact, many UK medical schools now incorporate elements of humanities in their curricula, often as part of the 'core', but also as student-selected modules which allow in-depth study.[42]
- *Widening participation.* It is Government policy to widen access to higher education. Historically, the stereotypical student entering medical school was male, middle class, educated in the independent sector and had achieved high grades in science subjects. All of this is changing, with an increasing proportion of female and mature students, and an intake from a broader and more eclectic academic base. New approaches to student selection, which attempt to identify qualities such as critical thinking, ethical awareness and emotional intelligence,[43] that may be predictive of more appropriate professional competencies are being introduced and evaluated.

It remains for the moment an article of faith as to whether these trends will change the culture of medicine.

Back to 'trust'

No claim could ever be made that courses on professionals and professionalism will guarantee that students will develop and maintain the 'correct' attitudes or demonstrate appropriate behaviour at qualification and for the rest of their careers, far less that they will bolster trust between patients and doctors. Nevertheless, education must provide some potential for change, although a significant shift is also required in the unwritten contract between society and medicine. Smith, for example, has written about this 'bogus contract', that is underpinned by unreal and unattainable expectations. He has argued the case for developing a contract that is more realistic, whereby the limitations of medicine are openly acknowledged by both the profession and the public. This, he argues, may lead to 'a much more honest, adult and comfortable relationship'.[44]

Ultimately, changes in policy and practice are more powerful drivers of change in education rather than the reverse.[17] The call for greater accountability and partnership, and the introduction of systems such as clinical governance and professional revalidation, which focus as much on who the doctor is and how they approach practice as on what they know and can do, mean that professional development will remain on the agenda of healthcare educators for the foreseeable future.[45]

- Until quite recently, what it means to be an authentic professional has been taken for granted in medical education.
- There is now an emphasis on what doctors should be, in contrast to what they should know or be able to do.
- Important components in the teaching of professionalism include medical ethics, communication, learning from errors, truthfulness, involving patients, and learning from communities.
- A correct expression of professionalism is a key factor contributing to a trusting doctor–patient relationship.

Acknowledgements

The author wishes to thank Reverend Bryan Vernon, Newcastle, for details of the ethics curriculum at Newcastle Medical School, Dr Annie Cushing, Barts & The London School of Medicine, for the empathy exercise, and Dr Gail Young, Newcastle, for helpful comments.

References

1   Calman K (1994) The profession of medicine. *BMJ.* **309**: 1140–3.
2   Cribb A and Bignold S (1999) Towards the reflexive medical school: the hidden curriculum and medical education research. *Stud Higher Educ.* **24**: 195–209.
3   Howe A (2002) Professional development in undergraduate medical curricula – the key to the door of a new culture? *Med Educ.* **36**: 353–9.
4   Stephenson A, Higgs R and Sugarman J (2001) Teaching professional development in medical schools. *Lancet.* **357**: 867–70.
5   British Medical Association (1995) *Core Values for the Medical Profession in the Twenty-First Century: conference report.* British Medical Association, London.
6   General Medical Council (2001) *Good Medical Practice.* General Medical Council, London.
7   Medical Professionalism Project (2002) Medical professionalism in the new millennium: a physician's charter. *Lancet.* **359**: 520–2.
8   American Board of Internal Medicine (2002) Medical professionalism in the new millennium: a physician's charter. *Ann Intern Med.* **136**: 243–6.
9   General Medical Council (1993) *Tomorrow's Doctors. Recommendations on undergraduate medical education.* General Medical Council, London.
10 General Medical Council (2002) *Tomorrow's Doctors.* General Medical Council, London.
11 American Board of Internal Medicine (1994) *Project Professionalism.* ABIM, Philadelphia, PA.

12 Cruess SR and Cruess SL (1997) Professionalism must be taught. *BMJ*. **315**: 1674–5.

13 Gordon J (2003) Fostering students' personal and professional development in medicine: a new framework for PPD. *Med Educ*. **37**: 341–9.

14 Arnold L (2002) Assessing professional behaviour: yesterday, today and tomorrow. *Acad Med*. **77**: 502–15.

15 Harden RM, Crosby JR and Davis MH (1999) Outcome-based education. Part 1. An introduction to outcome-based education. AMEE Guide No 14. *Med Teacher*. **21**: 7–14.

16 Hamilton JD (1999) Outcomes in medical education must be wide, long and deep. *Med Teacher*. **21**: 125–6.

17 Consensus Group of Teachers of Medical Ethics and Law in UK Medical Schools (1998) Teaching medical ethics and law within medical education: a model for the UK core curriculum. *J Med Ethics*. **24**: 188–92.

18 Nuffield Video Library in Medical Ethics and Law. *Informed Consent and Modern Medicine. Programme 3. Confidentiality and good hospital practice.*

19 Beauchamp T and Childress J (1983) *Principles of Biomedical Ethics.* Oxford University Press, Oxford.

20 Leape LL (1994) Error in medicine. *JAMA*. **272**: 1851–7.

21 Lester H and Tritter Q (2001) Medical error: a discussion of the medical construction of error and suggestions for reforms of medical education to decrease error. *Med Educ*. **35**: 855–61.

22 http://www.gmc-uk.org/standards/default.htm (accessed January 2003).

23 Silverman J, Kurtz S and Draper J (1998) *Skills for Communicating With Patients.* Radcliffe Medical Press, Oxford.

24 http://www.bristol-inquiry.org.uk/final_report (accessed January 2003).

25 Makoul G and Schofield T (1999) Communication teaching and assessment in medical education: an international consensus statement. *Patient Educ Counsel*. **137**: 191–5.

26 http://www.medicines-partnership.org/research–review/systematic-review (accessed January 2003).

27 Mercer SW and Reynolds WJ (2002) Empathy and the quality of care. *Br J Gen Pract*. **50/Quality Supplement**: S9–S12.

28 Spiro H, Curnen MGM, Peschel E and St James D (eds) (1993) *Empathy and the Practice of Medicine.* Yale University Press, New Haven, CT.

29 Novack DH, Suchman AL, Clark W, Epstein RM, Najberg E and Kaplan C (1997) Calibrating the physician. Personal awareness and effective patient care. *JAMA*. **278**: 502–9.

30 Coulter A (1999) Paternalism or partnership? *BMJ*. **319**: 719–20.

31 Towle A and Godolphin W (1999) Framework for teaching and learning informed shared decision making. *BMJ*. **319**: 766–71.

32 Spencer J, Blackmore D, Heard S *et al*. (2000) Patient-oriented learning: a review of the role of the patient in the education of medical students. *Med Educ*. **34**: 851–7.

33 Doyal L (2001) Closing the gap between professional teaching and practice. *BMJ*. **322**: 685–6.

34 Faulkner LR and Layton McCurdy R (2000) Teaching medical students social responsibility: the right thing to do. *Acad Med.* **75**: 346–50.

35 Russell A, van Teijlingen E , Lambert H and Stacy R (2003) *Social and Behavioural Sciences in Medical Education.* Department of Anthropology, University of Durham.

36 Spencer J (2002) What can general practice offer undergraduate medical education? In: J Harrison and T van Zwanenberg (eds) *GP Tomorrow* (2e). Radcliffe Medical Press, Oxford.

37 Spencer JA and Jordan RK (1999) Learner-centred approaches in medical education. *BMJ.* **318**: 1280–3.

38 McKegney CP (1989) Medical education: a neglectful and abusive family system. *Fam Med.* **21**: 452–7.

39 Newble D, Jolly B and Wakeford R (1994) *The Certification and Recertification of Doctors. Issues in the assessment of clinical competence.* Cambridge University Press, Cambridge.

40 Christopher DF, Harte K and George C (1996) The implementation of *Tomorrow's Doctors. Med Educ.* **36**: 282–7.

41 Philipp R, Baum M, Mawson A and Calman K (1999) *Humanities in Medicine. Beyond the millennium.* The Nuffield Trust, London.

42 Downie RS, Hendry RA, Macnaughton RJ and Smith BH (1997) Humanizing medicine: a special study module. *Med Educ.* **31**: 276–80.

43 http://www.acer.edu.au (accessed January 2003).

44 Smith R (2001) Why are doctors so unhappy? *BMJ.* **322**: 1073–4.

45 Spencer J (2000) Educating the coming generation. In: T van Zwanenberg and J Harrison (eds) *Clinical Governance in Primary Care.* Radcliffe Medical Press, Oxford.

CHAPTER 10

A profession's reputation

John Newton

> The purest treasure mortal times afford is spotless reputation; that
> away, men are but gilded loam or painted clay.
> (Shakespeare, Richard II, Act 1, Scene 1)

This chapter offers a sociological analysis of 'reputation' and its relationship
to our trust in professions. It is suggested that we have moved from a
'status'-based society where professional reputation was vital to a 'contract'-
based society where the State focuses instead on quantitative measures of
performance.

Introduction

A recent poll of listeners to the BBC Radio 4 *Today* programme found that doctors
and nurses topped a list of respected professions. Milkmen, computer pro-
grammers and farm workers were at the bottom of the list. This result might be
compared with an American survey conducted in 2001, in which respondents were
asked whether or not they would generally trust people in various different
professional groups (*see* Table 10.1).

Table 10.1   American propensity to trust

Professional group	Proportion of respondents generally prepared to trust members of specified profession (%)
Clergy	90
Teachers	88
Doctors	84
Police officers	78
...	...
Journalists	49
Members of Congress	42
Trade union leaders	37

What can be made of these rankings? What do they tell us about the reputation and trustworthiness of different occupations? 'One-off' surveys need to be treated with caution. For example, firemen (not 'firefighters'!) were fourth highest on the *Today* list, and this judgement might have had something to do with media coverage in the wake of the 9/11 terrorist attacks in America. A poll that was conducted following the UK firefighters' strike might give a quite different result. Even so, the *Today* poll does mirror findings of similar opinion surveys,[1] and similarities between the UK and American results (where both doctors and teachers, for example, are highly rated) are surely significant.

The results of these types of surveys raise a number of interesting questions. First, what is 'reputation' and how is it related to trust? Secondly, why are some occupations (or professions) regarded as more trustworthy than others? Thirdly, how stable are occupational reputations, and is there anything an occupation can do to sustain a good reputation, or to repair a damaged one?

Reputation and trust

The *Concise Oxford Dictionary of Current English*[2] defines reputation as 'what is generally said or believed about a person's or thing's character'. Now what is said or believed about a person or thing might not be true, or at least might be challenged. What is said or believed in one group or setting might not be the same as what is said or believed in another group or setting. And what is said might be quite different to what is believed!

Nonetheless, as a starting point this definition makes it clear that reputation is a quality which is formed through processes of social interaction and communication. Moreover, reputation is not exclusively a property of people. 'Things' such as products, organisations and occupations can have reputations, too.

According to Lang and Lang,[3] reputations vary along three dimensions (*see* Table 10.2).

Table 10.2   The three dimensions of reputation (from Lang and Lang[3])

1	Vertical – high reputation	Respect, authority and credibility is credited to the person
	Vertical – low reputation	The person is discredited
2	Lateral – limited extent	The person's reputation is limited to a particular neighbourhood or group of colleagues
	Lateral – wide extent	The person is well known in a wide public domain
3	Temporal – short duration	The person enjoys a short period of fame
	Temporal – enduring	The person benefits from a reputation that persists for many years

Occupations, like individuals, want to score highly along all three dimensions. They want to be well thought of, by as many people as possible, and for as long as possible – for reputation is a form of social capital, and a high reputation confers social and economic advantages.

In everyday social interaction, a person is more likely to gain the co-operation of another individual if he or she has a reputation for honesty or fair dealing. Similarly, an occupation with a longstanding reputation for, say, quality of service is more likely to retain and attract customers. Reputation provides customers with a guarantee of quality. This is particularly important if customers are not in a position to verify the quality of service themselves. In these circumstances, customers accept advice more on the basis of its source than on the basis of its content.

This last point suggests a strong relationship between reputation and trust. We tend to evaluate people and institutions in terms of prior notions and categories. These evaluations both shape the character of social interaction and influence the stability of social institutions. Reputation serves to order our social world. It shapes our perception of what a member of an occupation will be like and how he or she might act towards us. As such, it enables us to trust another 'by providing us with some information about the kind of person we are dealing with, before we have had a chance to have contact with that person'.[4] Thus reputation, allows people to trust others without deliberation or costly searching for evidence of capability or integrity. Trusting is a risky business, and knowing a trustee's reputation is one way of managing the risk. It is a particularly useful device for deciding about matters which cannot be settled immediately, but which depend on future events.

Establishing and sustaining a reputation for trustworthiness considerably enhances the way in which an occupation interacts with clients, other occupations and governments. Trustworthiness may above all else increase the amount of freedom from external regulation and control that is enjoyed by an occupation. If we trust an occupation, we allow its members to get on with the job. How can we explain, then, why some occupations are accorded different levels of trustworthiness?

Occupations and their reputations

The Standard Occupational Classification used by the Office for National Statistics, lists no less than 23 000 different occupational titles. However, only a minority of these become recognised as such by those employed in them and by the public at large. These socially recognised occupations usually form around specialised activities where those doing the work see some common interest in organising themselves. An early historical example of this type of occupational association was the medieval guild, which was formed to control entry to the occupation and to provide mutual aid and protection.

The development of industrial society tended to undermine the 'occupational principle' of work organisation[5] in favour of the 'administrative principle'. Work was organised in factories, and emphasis was placed on the design of tasks through the hierarchical division of waged labour. Trades and crafts, of course, persisted well into the industrial era. However, with the growth of bureaucratised work organisations, the specific tasks in which a person was engaged, and the skills allied to them, became less significant than the organisation in which the person was employed.[6] An important exception to this growing bureaucratisation of work was the emergence of middle-class professions in the mid- to late nineteenth century. It is these occupations that are of particular interest when considering reputation and trustworthiness.

The distinctiveness of the professions lies in the control that professionals have over the nature and conditions of the work compared with non-professionals – who are usually controlled by managers and supervisors. There are two aspects to professions' control over work. The first is autonomy – the freedom to make judgements and decisions without interference from anyone outside the profession. The second is self-regulation – the power of the occupation as a collective body to control education and training, to award licenses and to maintain standards of practice. It is interesting to consider what the conditions were in the mid- to late nineteenth century that allowed a number of occupations to become established as bodies that were aloof from the processes that were turning most workers into employees.

Most sociological analyses of professionalisation agree that a profession is established when the members of an occupation combine to control a market for their expertise, and when this is granted legitimacy by the State. Becoming a profession is an occupational strategy whose success depends on the following:

- possessing a body of knowledge which can be applied to practical affairs
- collective organisation
- striking a bargain with the State.

Therefore, in order to understand how professions earn, establish or are endowed with their reputations, we need to look at the social institutions in which knowledge is created, the institutions of the professions themselves, and the State institutions which allow professions to exercise their authority.

Professional knowledge is distinct both from everyday knowledge and from the 'know-how' that is involved in other occupations or trades. It is knowledge that Freidson calls *formal* knowledge (*see* Box 10.1).

Box 10.1   Formal knowledge

If there is a single concept by which the nature of formal knowledge can be characterized, the most appropriate is likely to be the rationalization (which) ... consists in the pervasive use of reason ... to gain the end of functional efficiency. ... Above all it is intimately associated with the rise of modern science and the application of the scientific method to technical and social probems.[7]

Formal knowledge, especially scientific knowledge as created and taught in universities, marks off professions and provides them with their basic credentials. However, professions are more than occupations whose members have university degrees. They are *organised* occupations whose members are influenced, moulded and controlled by their professional training and socialisation. However, this ability to regulate themselves depends crucially on the State granting them the licence to do so.

Why would the nineteenth-century *laissez-faire* State allow some occupations to become monopolies? The answer is that the successful occupations (i.e. those which achieved professional status) managed to convince powerful elites that it would be in the mutual interest of both the State and the occupation to strike a bargain. The occupation obtains jurisdiction over its expertise and can protect itself from occupational competitors, while the State obtains delivery of a much needed service and does not have to be concerned with regulating such matters itself. In clinching this bargain, reputation and trust play an important and self-reinforcing role. The aspiring occupation has to persuade the State that it can be entrusted to use its autonomy to further the interests of clients and society in general. However, it can only do this if it has already established a reputation.

Once it has been granted professional status, the occupation can proceed to enhance its reputation by all manner of displays. For example, the newly licensed Institute of Chartered Accountants in England and Wales (1880) acquired a prestigious site in the City of London on which it commissioned a building that would embody its new-found status. The editor of *The Accountant* proclaimed that 'As the new building arises so will the reputation of the profession gradually ascend in the public's estimation.'[8]

Unfortunately, there is no evidence to show whether the public did hold accountants in greater esteem after the building of their new headquarters, but this example does illustrate how reputation is partly a self-manufactured phenomenon. If reputation is what people say or believe about us, then this is by no means independent of what we persuade them to say or believe. Our reputation is to some extent in our own hands. Indeed, the history of professions shows that the occupations which have been most successful in establishing public trust through reputation are the ones which have used their knowledge base initially to create an occupational identity, and subsequently to gain a monopoly of the market for their expertise.

It is important not to neglect the knowledge base of the professional project. Professions earn their reputation in the first place because they offer something that is useful to society. With few exceptions we are all keen to live as long as possible, we all need to protect our possessions (property, wealth, etc.), and many of us are still concerned about our destiny beyond this life. On the basis of these enduring interests, and the ability of doctors, lawyers and priests to advise us on such matters, the professions of medicine, law and the clergy have emerged. Decorators and hairdressers have not sought such status, and it is unlikely that they would succeed in any such endeavour. This is because their skills do not reside in any formal knowledge, and also because we could all, if we wished, sort these things out ourselves, and could just about manage without them altogether. This is not to say that individual decorators and hairdressers do not have repu-tations – indeed, we frequently use recommendations based on evaluations of their competence or skill. The point is that there are some things which we regard as more central to human existence than others, and professions help us to minimise uncertainty in dealing with these issues (*see* Box 10.2).

Box 10.2   Professions are a means of coping with risk

The professional is our means of reducing uncertainty about important things that we cannot easily or economically verify ourselves.[9]

We are prepared to pay for professional judgement and knowledge because we trust the professionals, and our trust is partly a product of the attention that professions pay to their reputation.

However, the services that society sees as valuable are historically specific, as are the circumstances in which some groups come to monopolise the market for them. This means that the professions which are trusted today may not be trusted tomorrow. Social capital is more brittle than material forms of wealth.

Changing relationships between professions and society

By virtue of their occupational monopolies, their insulation from market forces and their ability to create and sustain a reputation for trustworthiness, the professions that were established in the mid- to late nineteenth century enjoyed considerable power and prestige in society. Some commentators have distinguished society that is based on specialised occupational expertise from the industrial society which preceded it (*see* Box 10.3).

Box 10.3   The professional society

The professional society is based on human capital created by education and enhanced by strategies of closure − that is, the exclusion of the unqualified.[10]

The 'professional society' is not simply a society that is dominated or ruled by professionals, but one in which the principle of trained expertise and selection by merit is paramount. In such a society, more and more occupations aspire to professional status and seek self-regulation of their work.

Professional society continued to thrive after the Second World War. Within the Welfare State, both the quantity and the quality of 'welfare' could be determined by professional judgement. This added to the power and authority of certain occupations.[11] Prior to the 1970s, apart from some critiques of the power of individual professions[12] there was very little questioning of the institutions and principles upon which the Welfare State was based.

However, in the late 1970s a combination of economic and political circumstances brought about a fundamental restructuring of State services. This in turn undermined the nineteenth-century 'bargain' between professions and the State. The nature of the restructuring has been described by Rudolf Klein[13] as a shift from a society based on status to one based on contract (*see* Table 10.3).

Essentially the status-based society is regarded as consisting of corporations (such as professions) that endow their members with status (or indeed reputation). These corporations operate under an arrangement with the State whereby they regulate their own affairs, exercise considerable autonomy in matters of professional judgement, and deal with clients on the basis of trust. The contract-based society, on the other hand, emphasises individualism, public regulation and external accountability.

Table 10.3   Characteristics of status-based and contract-based societies

Status-based society	Contract-based society
Corporatism	Individualism
Authority	Performance
Self-regulation	Public regulation
Autonomy	Accountability
Peers	Hierarchy
Trust	Review

Klein identified two major forces for change:

1 *laisser-faire economics*, which advocated the following:

   - the strict control of money supply
   - the breaking down of monopolies such as professions, and of restrictive practices enforced by trade unions
   - the injection of competition into the remaining parts of a much 'slimmer' public sector

2 *pressure to limit public expenditure* through the following:

   - managers exercising greater control over the resources committed by professional decisions
   - a greater concern with measurable 'outputs'.

Klein might have added 'consumerism' as a third force for change – that is, people having more knowledge, higher expectations and a greater readiness to challenge and complain.

The implications of a transformation from 'status' to 'contract' on trust have been well documented.[14] Using the distinction between social and economic exchange, Alan Fox has argued that, in the long term, a capitalist society progressively undermines trust in work roles and relationships.

- Social exchange involves 'favours that create diffuse future obligations (and) this requires trusting others to discharge those obligations'.
- Economic exchange, by contrast, stipulates precisely the nature and extent of each party's obligations.

Economic exchange does not rely on either party using its discretion, and it is associated with relationships that are based not on trust but on legally enforceable contracts.

Applying these principles to employment relations, Fox argues that the managers of capitalist enterprises, or indeed any organisation which is based on capitalist principles, try to minimise their dependence on employees by designing jobs which leave little room for discretion. The resulting pattern of relations is said to embody a low level of *institutionalised trust*. Managers do not trust employees to work with commitment. They put in place systems of close supervision to ensure satisfactory performance. Employees respond by refusing to invest any more effort than their contracts specify. If both parties continue like this, a self-perpetuating dynamic of mistrust is set in motion, characterised by calculating behaviour, opportunism and wariness. In fact, we end up with the opposite of the high-trust dynamic that formed the basis of Perkin's 'professional society' and Klein's 'status society'.

The changes in the Welfare State that were set in motion by governments from the late 1970s onward have lent little support to professionalism. In place of professionalism, the public sector has seen new structures of managerial control based on targets, outcomes and other 'deliverables' that are capable of being enumerated in contracts and standards, rather than the diffuse obligations that are inherent in a system of social exchange. We might wonder whether, if the new system leaves little room for trust, it also leaves little space for reputation.

Changing reputations

The new system of managing the welfare services has undermined not so much the reputation of any particular profession as the standing of professionalism in general. It has done this by appearing to rely more on audit, inspection and performance targets than on professional judgement. The 'new accountability', as Onora O'Neill describes these instruments,[15] has distorted the proper aims of professional work and has damaged institutionalised trust. Paradoxically, however, the professions which have been most subjected to the new accountability continue to enjoy high esteem in opinion surveys (such as the professions cited at the beginning of this chapter).

Perhaps this is because it is only the relationship between the state and the professions that has changed.

- The State has stopped trusting professionals, as is evidenced by the managerialist strategies which have imposed bureaucratic controls on them.
- The public, on the other hand, seems to hold professionals in the same high regard as it has always done, despite of a number of very well publicised failings in professional performance and conduct.

What is surprising is that a trail of recent scandals has not done irreparable damage to a range of professions, including the police, social workers and doctors. How have these professions managed to retain public confidence?

A great deal depends on the response that an organisation makes when its reputation is challenged. In very serious cases – the ones which become the subject of public inquiries – some judicial or quasi-judicial body makes recommendations with regard to what should be done to repair relationships with the organisation's stakeholders. A swift and publicly visible set of changes authorised by the organisation's chief executive or president is often sufficient to limit the damage and ward off further occurrences. The best interests of an organisation that is seeking to restore its reputation are not well served when a crisis or scandal is dealt with internally, and a statement is issued a long time after the event. If organisational or occupational reputations are at stake, honesty seems to be the best policy.[16]

To return to our opening quotation, the 'spotless reputation' that was cherished by the Duke of Norfolk in Shakespeare's *Richard II* is most likely to be established, sustained or rebuilt through openness with those whose confidence is being sought.

- Reputation involves the dimensions of strength (high or low), extent (limited or widespread) and duration (short-lived or enduring).
- Reputation is a significant factor in those situations where a client is unable to determine the quality of professional advice given for him- or herself, and therefore has little option but to trust the adviser.
- A high reputation will tend to increase the freedom from external regulation and control that a professional group can expect.
- The reputation of different occupational groups varies over time as the services that they supply are perceived as more or less valuable.
- Until the 1970s we lived in a 'professional' or 'status-based' society in which corporations could manage their own affairs, exercise considerable autonomy and professional judgement, and deal with their clients on the basis of trust and reputation.
- In the late 1970s, we saw a shift to a 'contract-based' society that emphasised individual performance, public regulation and external accountability. This change was driven by *laissez-faire* economics, pressure to limit public expenditure, and rising consumerism.
- In the new climate there is a preference for targets and measurable outcomes over the 'softer' qualities of reputation and trust. This new system of managing public services has tended to undermine trust in the professions in general.
- Ironically, although the State has stopped trusting professional groups, the level of public trust in professions such as medicine and nursing remains high.

References

1   MORI (2001) *Trust in Politicians, Civil Servants, etc.* http://www.mori.com/polls/trends/trust.shtml
2   (1995) *Concise Oxford Dictionary of Current English* (9e) Clarendon Press, Oxford.
3   Lang K and Lang GE (2001) Reputation. In: *International Encyclopedia of the Social and Behavioural Sciences. Volume 19.* Elsevier, Oxford.
4   Misztal BA (1996) *Trust in Modern Societies.* Polity Press, Cambridge.
5   Freidson E (1973) Professions and the occupational principle. In: E Freidson (ed.) *Professions and Their Prospects.* Sage, Beverley Hills, CA.
6   Watson TJ (1995) *Sociology, Work and Industry* (3e). Routledge, London.
7   Freidson E (1986) *Professional Powers.* University of Chicago Press, London.
8   Macdonald K (1995) *The Sociology of the Professions.* Sage, London.
9   Dingwall R (1996) *Professions and Social Order in a Global Society.* Plenary Presentation at the International Sociological Association (Working Group 02) Conference. Nottingham, September 1996.

10 Perkin H (1990) *The Rise of Professional Society: England since 1880.* Routledge, London.

11 Flynn R and Williams G (1997) *Contracting for Health: quasi markets and the National Health Service.* Oxford University Press, Oxford.

12 Illich I (1990) *Limits to Medicine. Medical nemesis: the expropriation of health.* Penguin, Harmondsworth.

13 Klein R (1990) From status to contract: the transformation of the British medical profession. In: HL L'Etang (ed.) *Health Care Provision Under Financial Constraint: a decade of change.* Royal Society of Medicine, London.

14 Fox A (1974) *Beyond Contract: work power and trust relations.* Faber, London.

15 O'Neill O (2002) *Spreading Suspicion.* BBC Reith Lectures 2002. A Question of Trust; http://www.bbc.co.uk/radio4

16 Irvine D (2001) The changing relationship between the public and the medical profession. *J R Soc Med.* **94**: 162–9.

CHAPTER 11

Learning from error

Jenny Firth-Cozens

It is one thing to show a man that he is in error, and another to put him in possession of truth.

(John Locke, 1690)

We often discover what *will* do, by finding out what will not do; and, probably, he who never made a mistake, never made a discovery.

(Samuel Smiles, 1859)

> This chapter describes how learning organisations increase both patient safety and professional job satisfaction.

The level of errors is reported to be high in healthcare. For example, the US Institute of Medicine, estimates that at least 44 000 people a year die as a result of medical error, and some studies suggest that the real number is twice that value. This has become a major concern for the media, the public, the Government and the professions. *An Organisation with a Memory*[1] was a Department of Health publication which focused on ways of recognising and reporting errors and learning from them so that their recurrence was made impossible or less likely. As a result of this document, a number of agencies have been created either to collect data on errors nationally and thus learn from them, or to assess doctors in difficulties.

My own interest in this area arose partly from my research on medical stress and mistakes[2,3] where doctors 'confessed' to incidents of poor care that they had given (some serious, and some in which the patient died as a result) which had often never been reported or previously discussed. The enduring guilt and anxiety about errors had been noted in previous studies,[4] and the need to confess was apparent from my conversations with others who had conducted similar surveys. The making of errors was clearly a major source of stress among doctors and probably among most healthcare staff.

My interest also arose from seeing young and not-so-young doctors who had been suspended for various reasons concerning errors or behaviours which had persisted for years but that had never been dealt with until suspension occurred. Failure to report these incidents earlier was leading to loss of doctors, and possibly also of patients, and to all the pain and distress that this involved for everyone concerned.

A considerable number of policy changes in the UK have led to better methods of collecting data on errors, but what is clearly needed to make these successful is to make learning from error the cultural norm. If we are to learn from error, we need to have accurate information about the errors that are being made, and this clearly requires a cultural change involving the development of sufficient trust to allow staff to report. This chapter will look first at a study of what people actually do when they see errors being committed or when they make them themselves,[5] and will then go on to consider how we can increase error reporting by developing higher levels of organisational trust.

What do staff do when they make or see an error?

In 2001, colleagues from the Northern and London Deaneries of Postgraduate Medicine and myself ran a series of focus groups for nurses and doctors of different grades to ask them what they actually did when they saw poor standards of care being given, or when they made an error themselves (*see* Box 11.1).[5] Interestingly, we could not persuade any of the four medical groups to discuss their own errors, although the nursing groups provided some examples. Therefore almost all of the results come from other people's errors or bad behaviour. Whether reporting these is more or less difficult than reporting one's own suboptimal care is an interesting research question that has yet to be studied.

Box 11.1   A senior nurse talks about learning from error[5]

I never checked the pump setting, I just whacked the thing in when I was doing a few other things and I suddenly looked at this guy's blood pressure and went 'Holy God!!', and that was it. The sweat was pouring off me, I thought I was going to be sick on the floor. He was absolutely fine, laying flat for a while but ... I remember this absolute battle-axe of a nursing officer coming up, and she said to me 'Every matron's made a mistake ... but how you feel is how everybody will feel when they've done it. But what have you learned from it?'

However serious the consequences, all of the groups described situations where reporting of errors would not take place (whether this was a single incident of poor care or bad behaviour). This was the most striking aspect of the group discussions (*see* Box 11.2).

Box 11.2   Errors that participants said they would *not* report

- Minor rather than major errors
- 'One-off' events rather than patterns of similar problems
- An error where the person making it was 'sorry' or showed insight
- Unavoidable error, where equipment might be to blame
- Bad behaviour, as opposed to error
- An 'otherwise good' doctor or nurse whom they would not wish to lose
- Unintentional errors

As a result of these consistently cited categories, silence about even very serious errors was ensured, and some errors which went unreported were described. However, there were slight differences between the groups. General practitioners appeared to be even less likely to report their concerns. This may have been partly due to the fact that they felt they could contain and remedy poor care within the practice, but it was also clearly due to their more acute need not to lose a doctor who would be difficult to replace. Senior nurses, overwhelmed by protocols which, if followed to the letter, could sometimes result in harm to patients, wondered whether action or inaction over a protocol was the error. Pre-registration house officers who had been clearly told by their consultants to report all mistakes to them said that they would never do this in practice: 'It's the worry that you won't get the support you need if you start complaining or pointing out errors.' The culture of silence had already enveloped them.

Bad behaviour was even more difficult to confront or report than poor clinical care, particularly in relation to doctors. This is partly due to enduring aspects of a macho medical culture and the question of what is acceptable within that culture. We were told that coming to work inebriated or seriously hung-over from the night before was not regarded as really unacceptable until doctors obtained their membership, at which point true professional behaviour was expected. Similarly, poor ways of interacting with patients and colleagues were tolerated or handled privately with enormous tact and sensitivity, rather than being addressed fully or reported.

There were examples of good practice, too, but these were rare. A consultant in Accident and Emergency reported the local learning that took place in their 'missed fracture' groups, where X-rays of fractures which had gone unnoticed were studied anonymously at regular intervals as a team learning session. Another consultant talked about the benefits of a ward-based 'time-out' in which care in general, including critical incidents, was discussed. Pre-registration house officers talked about the benefits of a group led by a nurse, discussing error and practice on the ward. A consultant talked about working with a colleague to address his poor behaviour over a period of years, and another had mentored a registrar who had problems with interpersonal skills. However, the point was made that these ways of addressing suboptimal care took up a considerable amount of time, which was becoming more and more difficult to find.

Barriers to change

There were other barriers to change (*see* Box 11.3) as well as a lack of time and resources to address errors properly, whether within the team or through the form-filling required to do this more systematically within the organisation. These barriers included an uncertainty about what was right or wrong, the difficulty of addressing problems in someone senior to oneself, and defining error too narrowly in the ways described above. The length of a contract was also given as a reason for not reporting someone's substandard care (both the short-term nature of medical and nursing training, and because someone would retire eventually) – for example, 'I thought, it's not a problem to me – I'm off soon' or 'All they did was say he'll retire soon'. However, a comparison was also made of the long-term 'here-for-the-duration' nature of the consultant's job, compared with the brief duration of many chief executives' time in post. For example, 'When you're talking about long-term problems that are to do with people's attitude and behaviour, you're the one who is going to be there for 20 years, needing effective working relationships with these people as colleagues. ... Deciding should we say something or not depends on what it might do to our working relationships' and 'NHS managers aren't always the right people to be looking at this. ... There's no point in having someone who is there for only a short time try and deal with a really difficult long-term problem.'

Box 11.3 Barriers to reporting

- Defining reportable errors too narrowly
- Length of contract provides excuses do do nothing
- The workload involved in reporting errors and the lack of resources to tackle this
- The persecutory ways in which error is handled – the culture of fear and the desire not to lose 'an otherwise good' nurse or doctor
- The fact that reporting has not been seen to bring about beneficial change
- Uncertainty about what is right or wrong

Some of these are likely to be – at least in part – defences against the very real anxiety about reporting error that was apparent in the groups. For many people it was fear that stopped them reporting. First, there was a lack of trust that the matter would be dealt with sensibly and sensitively (a dread of the 'dog-eat-dog' culture that currently exists in healthcare, or worries about losing an 'otherwise good' doctor or nurse who would be judged 'guilty until proven innocent'). Secondly, there was a fear that the individual who reported another's errors would suffer (that they would be ostracised, or would no longer get a good reference, and would be an 'easy scapegoat'). Fear was greatest among the nurses, particularly those at senior level, and among house officers, but to some extent all of the groups felt it.

This perceived culture of blame, shame and punishment prevents people from reporting the errors and behaviours of others, and almost certainly their own. It is strengthened by the wider societal culture of 'not telling tales' and, within healthcare, by stories and experiences of what will happen to a person if they do ('for about four months of that person's life it was made hell at work ... she just left'). This culture also contains the solidarity apparent in all of the groups that 'there but for the grace of God go I'. Such solidarity is likely to make the trust between colleagues greater, which will reduce the likelihood of their reporting incidents. In fact, what we see most clearly in this study, and in the culture that it describes, is a system where the culture of trust that is necessary for reporting error is almost entirely absent.

The context

What is the context in which people are able to take this trusting step? Lucien Leape describes the current emotional context very well:

> ... Patients and physicians ... live and interact in a culture characterized
> by anger, blame, guilt, fear, frustration, and distrust regarding health-
> care errors. The public has responded by escalating the punishment
> for error. Clinicians and some healthcare organizations generally have
> responded by suppression, stonewalling and cover-up.'[6]

This culture certainly provides strong incentives not to report error, and is one of
the primary barriers that needs to be tackled. However, this level of distrust by the
public has not always been present. Not so long ago doctors and health workers
enjoyed exceptionally high levels of trust, despite the fact that errors were unlikely
to be fewer in number than they are today. Errors went unacknowledged in what
has been termed 'a conspiracy of silence', although many whose errors harmed or
threatened patients suffered within this silence.[2] The reason for not reporting
errors then was not the culture of fear, but may rather have reflected the fact
that recognising and acknowledging a mistake which might well cause a patient
suffering or even death is to acknowledge the unthinkable – that one has harmed
someone whom one intended only to help. In an analysis of the psychodynamics
of safety at an oil refinery which had suffered two recent fires, Hirschhorn and
Young describe the ways in which dangerous environments are sometimes dealt
with psychologically – ways that create denial of the difficulties, that let staff feel
invulnerable and stop any thoughts of danger, and that use independent and risk-
taking 'heroes' to contain the anxiety that is felt by everyone, but who allow poor
work to continue as part of their macho risk-taking world.

Thinking about the emotional and psychological context of risk and safety is
immensely useful, and we can certainly learn from other industries, such as aviation.[7] However, we also need to remember that healthcare is an arena which,
I would suggest, creates far more anxiety about error than any other,[8] and thus it
is one where the recognition that harm has been caused to those we are trying to
help becomes much more difficult, while acknowledging error in others raises
anxiety about the very real possibility, or memory, of making a mistake oneself.
When considering how to build sufficient trust to enable us to learn from error, we
must be careful not to underestimate the level of this anxiety, and to acknowledge
and contain it as much as possible.[9]

The public will undoubtedly share this anxiety. After all, error is equally unthinkable to individuals who are about to put their own lives (if they are patients) or
those of their loved ones into the hands of others. Offering patients a deluge of
information about death rates, complications and substandard care, as has been
happening over the last few years, may seem like a way of involving them in
improvements in their care. However, if it is done without thought it can only
lead to the type of anger, punishment and rage that is so often seen nowadays if the
medical profession – trusted like a parent figure – then fails them. The stone-
walling and cover-up described by Leape follow as the doctors try to protect
themselves from both external blame and an internal acknowledgment of their own
human shortcomings. As O'Neill pointed out in her 2002 Reith Lectures,[10]
'Increasing transparency can produce a flood of unsorted information and mis-
information that provides little but confusion unless it can be sorted and assessed.
It may add to uncertainty rather than to trust'. Rather than increasing 'transparency', she suggests, we would do better to reduce deception. However, as we

have seen from the way in which waiting-list reporting has sometimes been economical with the truth, deception is likely to increase as the punishment for failure grows.

Another aspect of the context which affects the development or loss of trust involves the policy changes of the last decade or more. A growth in competition for the provision of healthcare is likely to have contributed to the cover-ups that Leape describes, while the reaching down by Government deep into healthcare itself is likely to begin to tarnish healthcare staff with the trust levels of politicians – not a welcome thought. In addition, a punitive, bullying approach by Government to management and clinicians is only likely to result in cover-ups. Finally, there is the ever-changing face of healthcare organisation. Such constant reorganisations disrupt relationships and networks, cause upheavals in established background assumptions, and thereby weaken trust which has sometimes taken years to build.

Trust and error making

In this context, the types of trust involved in learning from errors are complex and sometimes potentially conflicting. Trust is based on an underlying assumption of an implicit moral duty,[11] but here both trust to tell the truth and trust not to tell tales are involved, and they are rarely compatible. Similarly, we need trust to report our own errors, which is somewhat different to the trust that is needed to report the errors of others. In the case of reporting error, is this duty owed to the organisation who pays our salary and who wants to improve its safety record? Or is it owed to our colleagues with whom we experience solidarity, and whom we therefore want to protect from blame and punishment? Is it owed to current patients who have a right to know when things go wrong, or to future patients whose care we want to improve? In terms of the employing organisation, there needs to be trust by the management that they will have the full facts upon which to base decisions and improve quality, but there must also be reciprocal trust by the staff that management will not use the information to harm them. If reputation and its protection are an aspect of trust, what type of reputation is best protected? Are doctors protecting their reputations for honesty by owning up to errors and near-misses? Or are they protecting their reputations for providing the error-free care that the public expects? Historically, a considerable part of a doctor's power arose from the rise of science and his special knowledge, skills and mystery which resulted from this.[12] Therefore a recognition of error may be accompanied, in the short term at least, by a diminution of power, and we have seen this over the last decade as the imperfections of healthcare have become more apparent. I would suggest that in encouraging the development of the trust that is necessary to report errors and to learn from these errors in ways which will improve patient care, all of these facets of the trusting relationship need to be systematically taken into account, as well as the context in which those concerned perform their roles.

The rest of the chapter will discuss some of the ways in which trust can be developed and maintained so that organisations develop which can use error as an essential tool for learning and improving patient care.

Raising trust

Although some of the barriers to reporting error (e.g. problems with defining what is an error, uncertainty about what is right or wrong, and lack of time to complete forms) may be partly defensive against the anxiety that the recognition of error raises for staff, these barriers are nevertheless real. They are also among the first which need to be addressed, since when they are lowered we can see much more clearly what it is that still prevents people from reporting.

Clarifying accountability

There has been considerable talk of the 'no-blame' culture, which then became known as the 'just' culture,[1] and which our report[5] showed is clearly not believed in by many health service staff, overshadowed as it is by fear. There is no doubt that 'no blame' sits rather uncomfortably with 'accountability' (another byword of modern times which is rarely clarified). O'Neill, in her first 2002 Reith Lecture, questions the extent to which elaborate measures of accountability can ensure trust. There is no doubt that we have seen a meteoric rise in the development of protocols and of auditing them along with most other areas of both healthcare and public life in general. During this period it is true that, as O'Neill suggests, there is little evidence that trust has increased – rather the opposite. Nevertheless, I would still argue that, in aspects of life which involve real anxiety (and I have suggested that healthcare is certainly one of these), reducing aspects of uncertainty as much as possible, particularly in terms of role and responsibilities, is an important step. Brittain and Langill[13] describe the way in which their organisation did this by a process of outlining in detail the accountability and authority of employees and managers, the first assumption of which was that 'good working relationships require trust, and trust requires clarity of role definition'.

Clarification of accountability will be one step towards increasing people's understanding of what is error and what is acceptable behaviour. For example, in our study[5] it became apparent that young doctors coming to work under the influence of alcohol was not a situation that was regarded as totally unacceptable, but rather it was viewed as something that most people grew out of in time. Intoxicated doctors were sent home, but they were not reported. Such a misconception would be an easy place to start the process of defining which behaviours are not to be tolerated. In this way, staff with potential or real drink problems can be helped to overcome them. Another place where we could begin to clarify accountability is to emphasise that not reporting errors because our contract (or that of the error maker) is about to end is unacceptable. Staff need to understand that every error counts positively towards learning.

Organisational rewards must be directed towards the growth of error reporting, followed by learning and change, followed by rewards for demonstrated improvements in patient care.

Systems for gathering data

Emphasising the importance of recognising and collecting data on 'near-misses' as well as everything beyond them may help to show that 'trivial' or non-harmful incidents can still lead to valuable learning. Training staff in what is a near-miss, and what to do when they either have or see one, is another useful area in which to begin developing the organisation towards learning, since it involves errors which are not associated with the anxiety which arises from actually harming patients. However, whether errors cause harm or not, it is vital that systems for collecting the data, analysing it within the team or elsewhere, and learning lessons from it are made as streamlined and straightforward as possible, and that regular time is set aside for this activity.

The final essential step in increasing trust in this area is to ensure that change takes place as a result of the reporting activity. Managers and clinical staff must join together to make such change a priority, and to monitor its benefits carefully and publicise what has been done. Not following through on error reporting can be interpreted as demonstrating contempt for the real difficulties it involves for staff, and the efforts that they have made to overcome these obstacles.

These are the key organisational steps involved in raising levels of trust. However, none of these steps will be successful without leaders who are personally capable of gaining and maintaining the trust of their staff. This was clearly demonstrated by a study[14] which related team functioning to medication errors. It was found that good teams reported making more errors than poor teams – a result that only made sense when the further finding emerged that poor teams had more authoritarian leaders!

Better leadership

Of course, some people will find it easier to trust their leaders than others. A number of studies have shown that individual differences in the propensity to trust are considerable.[15] There is not much that can be done about this, apart from recognising that gaining the trust of a few brave souls may not imply that the rest are ready to reveal all. More important, therefore, is the research which demonstrates the characteristics of those who must be trusted if a learning organisation is to be created – characteristics which increase the perceived trustworthiness of leaders, whether they are managers or clinicians.

Within aviation, the training of leaders who are able to listen to others and who understand the nature of human error, the part played by stress and fatigue in error making, and the importance of two-way communication and monitoring[7,16] has been developed in response to terrible safety blunders in the past. A review of the characteristics of those who are trusted[17] revealed three attributes which appear across most of the literature – if they are to be trusted, leaders must have ability, benevolence and integrity.

In encouraging a climate of trust for reporting errors, I would suggest that one of the most important *abilities* to possess is an ability to admit openly to one's own errors. Trusting behaviours are necessary in relationships where power is unevenly distributed, as in the case of leaders and their staff. Gathering information about what those staff have done wrong is bound to increase the unevenness of power, whereas managers acknowledging their own mistakes is likely to balance things more evenly and thus to increase the likelihood of admissions of error in the future. Other crucial abilities involve listening skills, being able to provide a good, clear rationale for the need for error reporting and learning, and being able to follow through on the necessary changes.

Benevolence involves the appearance of wanting to do the best by one's staff, beyond one's own self-protection or profit. Within this area, benevolence involves the necessary recognition of the difficulties of clinical care, the stress and heavy workload that many face,[18] and the real anxiety that is involved in error making. Providing training in risk management and safety, and time to gather data and learn lessons from it, would all be essential steps in establishing that the difficulties are understood. Staff need to believe that their leaders intend the best for them and their patients, and demonstrating this is important. For example, where the media are involved in reporting an adverse incident, the leader has an opportunity to stand by his or her staff, their dedication and the excellence of their work almost all of the time. Another example would involve the leader being regularly seen at the coal-face so that he or she can experience directly the difficulties and anxieties of both staff and patients.

Integrity stands back-to-back with benevolence. It needs to be clear to those who trust that the trustee has values and principles and stands by them. Keeping one's word that errors will be treated non-punitively so long as safety protocols or agreed responsibilities have been adhered to would be one example of this. Within organisations such as Nissan, integrity is regarded as absolutely essential to the maintenance of quality – for once a manager allows something poor to pass through the system because of some expediency, trust is lost.[19] The characteristics of benevolence and integrity can be a real challenge to leaders who are given two conflicting roles by Government – to show ever greater efficiency while at the same time increasing the quality of care. Unless these characteristics of good leadership are in turn demonstrated to healthcare managers by those who control them, they are going to find it particularly difficult to have the capability to treat their staff in ways which will increase their trust.

Conclusions

This chapter has demonstrated the difficulties that staff experience with regard to reporting of errors, and thus the potential barriers to creating a learning organisation. It has outlined some of the ways in which these can be overcome and good leaders can take them forward as a process of organisational development. Most importantly, it has demonstrated the complexity of trust in this area – something which needs to be borne in mind constantly as steps are taken systematically to increase and maintain trust which will be sufficient to overcome the anxieties of staff about reporting when things go wrong.

- Medical errors are a frequent, daily occurrence.
- Professionals who make errors feel both stressed and guilty.
- A culture for reporting errors must be based on trust, not blame.
- Within teams, clarity of roles builds trust.
- Teams also need good leadership that is based on ability, benevolence and integrity.
- Learning organisations develop by reflecting on errors and changing behaviours appropriately.

References

1   Department of Health (2000) *An Organisation With a Memory: Report of the Expert Group on Learning from Adverse Events in the NHS.* Department of Health, London.

2   Firth-Cozens J and Greenhalgh J (1997) Doctors' perceptions of the links between stress and lowered clinical care. *Soc Sci Med.* **44**: 1017–22.

3   Firth-Cozens J (2001) Interventions to improve physicians' well-being and patient care. *Soc Sci Med.* **52**: 215–22.

4   Mizrahi T (1984) Managing medical mistakes: ideology, insularity and accountability among internists-in-training. *Soc Sci Med.* **19**: 135–46.

5   Firth-Cozens J, Redfern N and Moss F (2001) *Confronting Errors in Patient Care.* Department of Health, London; www.publichealth.bham.ac.uk/psrp/pdf

6   Leape LL, Woods DD, Hatlie MH *et al.* (1998) Promoting patient safety by preventing medical error. *JAMA.* **280**: 1444.

7   Helmreich RL (2000) On error management: lessons from aviation. *BMJ.* **320**: 781–5.

8   Firth-Cozens J (2002) Anxiety as a barrier to risk management. *Qual Safety Health Care.* **11**: 115.

9   Menzies-Lyth I (1988) *Containing Anxiety in Institutions: selected essays.* Free Association Books, London.

10 O'Neill O (2002) *Lecture 1: spreading suspicion.* BBC Reith Lectures, London.

11 Hosmer LT (1995) Trust: the connecting link between organizational theory and philosophical ethics. *Acad Manag Rev.* **20**: 379–403.

12 McCullough LB (ed.) (1998) *John Gregory's Writings on Medical Ethics and Philosophy of Medicine.* Kluwer Academic Publishers, Dordrecht.

13 Brittain B and Langill G (1997) Structuring the design and implementation of leadership and teamwork for program management. *Healthcare Manag Forum.* **10**: 50–52.

14 Edmondson AC (1996) Learning from mistakes is easier said than done: group and organizational influences on the detection and correction of human error. *J Appl Behav Sci.* **32**: 5–28.

15 Hofstede G (1980) Motivation, leadership and organization: do American theories apply abroad? *Organiz Dynamics.* **9**: 42–63.

16 Firth-Cozens J and Mowbray D (2001) Leadership and the quality of care. *Qual Health Care.* **10** (**Supplement II**): 7.

17 Mayer RC, Davis JH and Schoorman FD (1995) An integrative model of organizational trust. *Acad Manag Rev.* **20**: 709–34.

18 Wall TD, Bolden RI, Borril CS *et al.* (1997) Minor psychiatric disorder in NHS trust staff: occupational and gender differences. *Br J Psychiatry.* **171**: 519–23.

19 Binney G and Williams C (1997) *Leaning Into the Future: changing the way people change organizations.* Nicholas Brealey Publishing, London.

CHAPTER 12

Sharing information with patients

Di Jelley and Caron Walker

GP: Well, Mrs S, your cholesterol level is a bit high – we can either start drug treatment straightaway or you could try working hard to alter your diet and see if we can get it down that way.

Mrs S: I don't know what to think – you're the doctor – surely you know best ...

This chapter describes examples of sharing information with patients, and explores what needs to be done to make such sharing effective. Sharing information and decision making represents a fundamental shift in the traditional relationship between patient and professional. Professionals need to change their attitudes and develop appropriate skills.

Introduction

'The doctor knows best'. Until perhaps ten years ago, this statement would have summed up the basic tenor of most doctor–patient interactions. Students went to medical school to learn how to diagnose and treat disease, and this educational model also underpinned their postgraduate medical training. They gradually acquired the skills and knowledge to become competent in their chosen speciality, but there was little formal training in the process of consulting. A good 'bedside manner' was acknowledged as a characteristic of high-quality care, but this was in terms of thoughtful and sensitive explanations of diagnostic findings and treatment plans, rather than actively involving the patient in decisions. Doctors told patients their recommended course of action, and patients expected to be told what was to be done to them. Bad news was often communicated initially to relatives, who would then decide with the doctor exactly how much information the patient should be given.

In recent years there has been a gradual shift in the belief systems which underpinned these behaviours – a change that perhaps reflects the altering relationship between the professions, the public and the State. For example, it has been shown that doctors are not always able to regulate members of their own profession, and their authority has been called into question. The public has begun to ask whether they can trust the doctor who is treating them. Patients want and need to trust their doctors, but they now want to do this from a position of mutual understanding and joint decision making. For this reason, sharing information with patients in an accessible and meaningful way may be of critical importance to the future relationship between doctors and their patients.

Information sharing: some key examples
Data Protection Act: access to medical records

General practitioners in the UK hold a considerable amount of information about their patients. There are hand-written or computer-recorded consultation summaries, letters between primary and secondary care services, test results and copies of insurance and employment reports. Since the 1992 Data Protection Act, patients have been entitled to request and read their medical records, yet experience suggests that few patients request access to their records unless they are checking a specific query. In any case, medical records are often difficult for patients to understand, because of poor handwriting and the use of abbreviations and medical terminology. Simply giving patients the right to inspect their records does not necessarily increase the amount of useful personal health information that is available to them. Other mechanisms are needed, some of which have been in place for a long time, while others are new initiatives.

Giving patients their records to read before they see the doctor

Since 1983, Baldry and colleagues[1] in a group practice in London have been giving patients their records to hold before they go in to see the doctor or nurse. Most of these patients take the opportunity to read their notes, but any new 'bad news' is filed elsewhere until it has been discussed with the patient. Letters or reports containing significant third-party information (e.g. child protection case conference reports) are also filed separately from the main records. In rare instances, records have been withheld from severely disturbed patients. All of the doctors make time to go through the records with any patients who request help in understanding what has been written about them. Errors of fact have been corrected as necessary, and there have been few instances of patient distress or disagreement.

The group of patients who expressed most concerns after seeing their records were those with mental health problems. They often found the labelling of their illness and the accounts of their behaviour when unwell very distressing to read. This issue is currently being addressed in a Department of Health pilot study. Most patients in a waiting-room survey indicated that access to their records had helped to break down barriers between themselves and their doctors. They felt that the process was reassuring, helpful and informative. The overall assessment of sharing records openly with patients in this way was very positive – putting a premium on accuracy and clarity in the written record and encouraging honesty. Now the challenge is how to maintain this openness of access to records as the practice becomes paperless and all records are stored on computer. One wonders why such an easy way of providing patients with access to their records has not been adopted more widely.

Shared electronic patient records

The electronic patient record (EPR)[2] has been used experimentally in a few pilot sites over the past five years. Medical records are carefully reviewed and all relevant information is transferred to a single electronic record that can be viewed by the patient in the surgery or at home. Primary and secondary care services can also view the same record. The main advantage to patients is that they do not have to keep repeating biographical data when they are referred to secondary care. They can also keep an accurate track of appointments and test results. As part of a pilot project, patients have also had ready access to an information support worker who could help them to find and interpret the information in their record. It is unlikely that such support could ever be funded on a national scale if and when the EPR becomes standard for all patients. However, this may be the only way for some groups of patients to access the written word.

Patient-held records

Obstetric and paediatric services have led the way with patient-held records, which are also used widely in developing countries. Patient-held antenatal or child-health record cards have been the norm in some units for more than two decades, and there have been a number of formal evaluations. Stevens describes the use of a patient-held record in paediatric oncology in which current treatment, test results and consultation reports are recorded.[3] These shared records have been shown to save time, reduce errors in dosage scheduling, and promote continuity of care between different treatment sites such as outpatients, casualty and primary care. There is also a reduction in paper correspondence between sites, and the record acts as an educational resource for families. However, a randomised controlled trial in which adult cancer patients were given copies of their own records failed to find any differences between the two groups in terms of patient satisfaction, participation in care or quality of life.[4] Jones and colleagues[5] have described a study in which patients were provided with an integrated medical and dental patient-held record. Patients valued seeing their own records – nearly a third of patients identified inaccuracies and omissions – and dentists were enthusiastic about having more ready access to patients' medical records.

Copying letters to patients

Much information about an individual's health is contained in the letters which pass between primary and secondary care services, but it has never been routine practice to share these letters with patients. A number of small studies and anecdotal reports suggest that patients do appreciate receiving copies of clinical correspondence that is written about them. Scott and colleagues[6] examined the effects of providing recordings or written summaries of their consultations to people with cancer. They found that adult cancer patients and their families found this information useful and helpful. In contrast, a randomised controlled trial in which GP referral letters were copied to patients showed no difference between the two groups in terms of attendance rates at outpatients. However, no other indices of satisfaction were examined.[7]

We have conducted two studies on this topic based in a number of practices in North-East England. Both of the studies have shown that patients welcomed receiving a copy of their referral letter. They stated that it made them feel better prepared for the clinic appointment and better informed about what was happening to them. There was a clear message that having a copy of the letter, especially for more complex problems, allowed patients to reflect on what had been said in the consultation and to discuss their concerns with family and friends if necessary. Almost all of the patients felt that copying letters should become routine practice.

However, local general practitioners and consultants who were surveyed in the same study had concerns about the process. They felt that although patients might benefit from more open sharing of information, there would be considerable difficulties in writing letters that were both useful and understandable to patients and at the same time sufficiently informative for colleagues. There was a feeling that 'dumbing down' the content of letters in order to make them accessible to patients would reduce their professional quality. There were also concerns that raising the possibility of tentative but serious diagnosis in a letter might frighten patients unnecessarily, and that useful but sensitive information such as a history of alcohol abuse or domestic violence might be excluded from letters being copied to the patient. There was also a strong belief that the process would significantly increase workload.[8,9]

The positive views of patients in these studies encouraged us to start copying referral letters to our patients as a matter of routine in 2001. A third study now in progress confirms patients' positive response to the process, and shows clearly that patients' anxiety levels were not increased further by receiving copy letters, but rather they appreciated knowing exactly why they were being referred. All doctors in the practice, including locums and GP registrars, have adopted this policy, and between 80% and 90% of all letters are now sent to patients by post. A few patients refuse the offer of a copy letter, and occasionally the doctor decides not to send one (e.g. when third-party information is a prominent feature, or in some cases of mental illness). The increase in workload for our doctors has been minimal (the occasional telephone query about a letter, or a timely reminder that the letter has not actually been written!). Adapting to a writing style that is both accessible to patients and informative to hospital colleagues has also not been difficult. However, there is an administrative cost in terms of both time and resources that will need to be recognised when 'letters between clinicians about an individual patient's care will be copied to the patient as of right' in 2004 as stated in the NHS Plan.[10]

Larger and more systematic studies with robust outcome indicators will be needed to confirm the benefits of this shift towards more open sharing of information and decision making with patients. However, the above studies, as well as the findings from other small studies, all suggest that patients welcome this changing process. A review by Guadagnoli and Ward[11] of patient participation in decision making found that patients want to be involved in treatment decisions, especially if alternative treatments are available. There was no clear evidence of the benefits of this involvement, but the authors argue that patient participation is justified 'on humane grounds alone'. Some of the major challenges facing the health service are how to facilitate this process, how to provide patients with accessible and helpful information, and how to involve them effectively in decision making about their health and healthcare. There are a number of ways in which this could be done.

Sharing information effectively: what needs to be done to make it work?

General health information

The central importance of providing accessible information for patients was addressed in a recent Department of Health strategy document,[12] in which it is argued that information sources for patients must be clearly signposted, and that the information provided must be reliable, clear and intelligible. A number of organisations, including the King's Fund, have published a guide to help anyone who is producing information for patients.[13] Our research indicates that patients and carers, especially those with long-term health problems, are usually quite clear what they want to know about their illness and its treatment.[9]

Advances in information technology have great potential to improve the quality and accessibility of health service information, and there are national initiatives to increase access to the Internet for deprived or isolated communities. Health professionals need to be able to direct patients to sources of good-quality consumer health information, identifying reliable websites. Jadad[14] argues that the Internet provides opportunities to enhance partnerships between clinicians and patients, but this requires a concordance of values between the information providers and users.

Personal health information

If we consider the specific context of clinical correspondence being sent to patients, a number of important issues emerge. These will need to be addressed so that copied letters can become a useful tool for enhancing communication with all patients.

Electronic information and communication

Sending paper copies of letters to patients may be just a temporary stage in the evolution of information sharing between doctors and patients. The advent of the electronic patient record and the possibility of establishing direct email contact between patients and clinicians may further alter the nature of this changing relationship. Pal[15] describes the use of email to elicit and respond to patient queries, and believes that this can be a safe and useful enhancement of normal communication tools if it is appropriately monitored.

Access for patients with reading difficulties

There are four groups of patients for whom access to the written word may be difficult, and whose specific needs must be addressed. These are patients with visual impairment, learning disabilities or deafness, and those who do not have English as their first language. The Disability Discrimination Act 1995 and the

Race Relations Act 2000 provide the legal framework for preventing service providers from discriminating against such patients, and require them to provide information in an accessible form. This may mean providing information in the usual alternative formats – that is, large print, tape or Braille (which is used by only a minority of the visually impaired population) – but for some this may still render the information inaccessible. For example, someone with a visual impairment might want the information to be provided on a compact disc which can be listened to, or on one with text which can be enlarged on their own computer. Alternatively, someone with a learning disability might need their information to be presented in diagrammatic form, such as drawings or symbols. Doctors may need to store a bank of suitable photographs in their computer, which can then be used in letters and documents.

This is where voluntary organisations have a crucial role to play. Organisations for disabled people and ethnic minorities have the expertise to provide accessible information for their members. Therefore, the health service needs to work with them to ensure that accessible information is provided for all patients.

Use of appropriate language

Information that is sent to patients must be understandable at a level that corresponds to average reading ability in the local community. The Plain English Campaign has produced a guide to help doctors to make letters and medical information clearer for patients. It has also published a glossary of medical terms translated into language that everyone can understand.[16] Our experience of copying letters to patients is that remarkably few patients request explanations of letters from their doctors. However, many seek help from relatives or friends, or turn to other sources of written or electronic information. In our most recent survey the patients said that they understood the letters they received, but this has not yet been evaluated objectively.[9]

Consent and confidentiality

Information sharing is not a one-way process. If it is to be of benefit, it must be accepted, wanted and understood by patients. Patients have a right to know about their illnesses and proposed treatments. Importantly, they also have a right not to know, and not to have to make decisions about treatment options if they do not want to. Thus any opening up of communication with patients must be on the basis of informed consent, and that consent must be revisited in each illness episode. An individual who is happy to receive a copy of their referral letter for a hip joint replacement might not feel the same way about a referral for counselling concerning past abuse.

There are also important issues relating to confidentiality. In some areas, especially in large cities, patients' addresses may change frequently and letters may go astray or to the wrong address. In some households the intended recipient may not open letters, and letters containing sensitive information may be lost or mislaid. Asking the patient to collect the letter from the surgery or hospital puts pressure on already over-burdened receptionists or secretaries to ascertain the correct identity of every patient who requests their copy letter. Ultimately, it must be expected that errors will occur. This is the inevitable price of increased openness, and health professionals will need to be supported in dealing with the consequences of any such mistakes.

Letters that help as well as inform the patient

There is some evidence from work with psychiatric patients that letters can be used not only to impart information but also to encourage reflection and learning by the patient. White and Epston[17] build on the theory that 'knowledge is power' and that patients can thus be empowered by information which is provided in an accessible yet challenging way. The letter from the outpatient consultation is written to the patient and copied to the referring physician. This letter is not simply a record of the interview, but is written in a style that is designed to enhance key points where decisions needed to be made or where new actions or choices were discussed. Direct questions may be asked in the letter to stimulate reflection by the patient before the next meeting. This approach to letter writing has not been applied in a primary care setting, but as sharing becomes more widely adopted, the role of the enhanced 'therapeutic' letter merits further exploration.

Involving patients in decision making

Information that is shared with patients must not only be readable and accurate, but may also increasingly need to support patients in making choices. The shift away from a paternalistic consulting style towards one that is more patient-centred will often lead the clinician to offer the patient a range of treatment options. For example, do they want physiotherapy for their knee pain or would they prefer medication or an injection? Do they feel happy about antidepressant medication or would they prefer referral to a counsellor or regular review in the surgery? The advance of evidence-based practice has provided some clear guidance on best practice, but it has also highlighted the many areas where there is no clear evidence to underpin clinical decision making. In these situations, patients are increasingly being given a choice. Some reject this overture, adopting the stance of 'Don't ask me, I'm not the doctor', but others seem keen to consider the potential of different management options.

There is now a considerable body of literature supporting patient involvement in decision making. O'Connor and colleagues[18] have recently summarised the findings of studies on decision aids for patients and found that these can improve knowledge, reduce decisional conflict and increase active involvement in decision making. Coulter and colleagues[19] reviewed some of the information that is available to patients to support their involvement in treatment decisions. They found that such information materials often omit relevant data, fail to give a balanced view of the effectiveness of different treatments, and ignore uncertainties. They concluded that patients should be involved in the production and testing of any such materials. Patients do have access to a wide variety of information sources of variable quality, and many will use these when considering treatment choices. Clinicians now have an additional pastoral role in guiding and supporting patients through this often difficult decision-making process.

Sharing risk with patients

Perhaps the most difficult aspect of this new challenge for clinicians is the effective sharing of decisions involving risk. Informed choice for patients must be based on adequate information covering the options, risks and benefits. Doctors who are helping patients to assess these criteria have a responsibility to check the patient's understanding of the issues involved. Most critically, patients need to be clear that there are circumstances where there is considerable debate among clinicians about the relative effectiveness of different treatments. Doctors will need to find a way of sharing these uncertainties with their patients.

Edwards and Elwyn[20] have highlighted the variety of information which is given to consumers and the ethical issues that this raises. They argue that patients need information to be presented in a balanced way, and that they need professionals who do not manipulate them towards specific choices. There are training implications here for all health professionals on how to present information in a balanced way, and how to step back from using their inherent power in the consultation to influence patient choice when a range of alternative options is being considered. The aim is to make choices, rather than one preferred path, explicit to the patient. This observation – that more open communication with patients requires changes in consulting style – leads us on to the final section in this chapter.

Information sharing and shifting roles: the challenges ahead

Information sharing is but one part of a broader picture – it is one aspect of the larger project of rebuilding trust in the context of the doctor–patient relationship. Sharing uncertainty and risk with patients, sending them copies of clinical letters written about them, and supporting them in making decisions about treatment options all alter the prevailing dynamic of the doctor–patient relationship that has been with us for so many years. The events of the last five years have undermined the foundations upon which 'blind' trust between clinicians and patients was built. The new era of 'enlightened' trust requires a change in professional attitudes and the development of new skills. Information sharing cannot take place in a vacuum – there are key areas that will have to underpin its successful implementation.

Patient partnership: what does it really mean?

Traditionally, the main boundary in healthcare provision has been that between doctor and patient, and many health professionals and patients would be the first to recognise that this relationship between doctor and patient has never been an easy one. Until recently, the doctor was the one who had the knowledge, and it was difficult for patients to gain access to it. Bacon famously said that 'knowledge itself is power', and in the mind of the patient this rang true. Their doctor had power by virtue of his or her knowledge, and power is not easily relinquished, for it is acknowledged that 'social power is an integral aspect of the daily working lives of professionals'.[21]

The mantra of 'partnership' has been increasingly promoted in policy documents as a means of shifting this balance of power away from professionals and towards patients. Defining what is meant by the concept of partnership is not an easy task, because the word 'partnership' means different things to different people. In its broadest sense, working in partnership can relate to organisations or individuals working together or acting jointly.[22] It could be a core organisational principle, such as an agreement to share information with patients. However, it could also reflect an attitude or stance that there needs to be a fundamental shift of power away from the professional.[23]

Much of the debate about the need for partnership has focused on the need for collaborative working between professionals, rather than between professionals and patients. Governments (of all persuasions) have placed an emphasis on the need for different agencies to work together to develop more integrated health and social care provision.[24] There are barriers to closer working between professionals, and these are often manifested by a degree of rivalry. Bringing patients and carers into this equation merely adds to the complexity of these relationships.

Nevertheless, from all sides partnership and collaborative working are considered to be 'a good thing'. This view rests on the expectation of an increase in choice and control for patients. In primary care, this has been reflected in a substantial shift towards greater patient involvement in the decision-making process with regard to their healthcare. It is also seen as part of a wider aim of achieving a greater degree of equality between patients and healthcare professionals. However, there is still suspicion among patients that real choice may be a mirage, because health professionals continue to be the gatekeepers of information, knowledge and services. Opening the gate is perceived as a threat to both profession and professionalism.

Recognising and acknowledging these tensions – between professionals, and between professionals and patients – may be the best way forward for developing a meaningful partnership between patients and doctors. Dissent could be a major factor in relationships between professionals and users of services. Dale proposes that a partnership should be:

> a working relationship where the partners use negotiation and joint decision making and resolve differences of opinion and disagreement, in order to reach some kind of shared perspective or jointly agreed decision on issues of mutual concern.[25]

The expert patient

Providing patients with the means and skills to access both personal and more general health information alters the balance of power in the doctor–patient relationship. The doctor may not ' know best', and particularly in the context of rare conditions he or she may know considerably less than the patient. An extension of 'patient partnership' casts patients as experts who can educate their clinicians. There are already reports of the successful involvement of patients as expert resources, rather than passive tools, in the education of medical students.[26] There have been exciting initiatives in Germany where patients have been educated in the care of their hypertension and diabetes to the extent that they start, stop and change their medication without guidance from their physicians. They achieve excellent levels of disease control as a result.[27]

Chambers has written a practical guide on how to increase the effective involvement of patients in the planning and delivery of their healthcare. She emphasises how changing patient expectations are driving more effective partnerships with healthcare professionals.[28] However, it is not only patients who will have to change if this relationship is to be sustained and nurtured.

Changing attitudes, developing skills

Healthcare professionals in all fields have been trained to assess, advise and administer treatments. The basic assumption is that our training equips us to make decisions on behalf of our patients. Even when we have been unsure, we have rarely shared this uncertainty with the patient. Information sharing challenges this basic assumption and requires us to share our decision making with patients. If we are referring a patient with a breast lump to hospital, we must discuss our concerns and our assessment of the risk of a serious outcome with the patient before they receive their copy letter. If we are referring a patient with depression to the practice counsellor, we must clarify whether they willingly agree to information on past abuse being included in the letter. Similarly, the patient who has been seen in the outpatient clinic with a new diagnosis of leukaemia or angina will need to have the diagnosis and management explained to them before they receive a copy of the clinic letter. Open sharing of information drives better consulting, and should also highlight the need for a lifelong commitment to regular consultation skills training.

Conclusion

Information sharing is a powerful tool that both clinicians and patients have only just begun to use effectively. It is a tool that can empower patients, allowing them to take part in decisions that affect their health and healthcare, and it drives the doctor–patient relationship away from paternalism towards a more equal partnership. Information sharing affects clinicians in other ways, challenging them to face their uncertainties. This means acknowledging the lack of an evidence base for much of what they do, and being open about limitations when treatment options are being discussed. Openness in all aspects of doctor–patient communication will drive better and more patient-centred consulting, and should lead to greater patient satisfaction.

Sharing our beliefs, concerns and uncertainties with patients, as they share theirs with us, could provide a basis from which the process of rebuilding trust can proceed.

- There are already examples of information sharing, such as shared electronic patient records, patient-held records, and copying of referral letters.
- Patients want more information about health in general and about their own health in particular, and they value information sharing and shared decision making.
- There are practical issues that need to be addressed, such as the use of appropriate language, access for those with reading difficulties, and consent and confidentiality.
- True patient partnership requires professionals to cede some of their power.

Acknowledgements

The authors of this chapter are indebted to Lindsey Graham for use of the excellent bibliography, *Preparing Professionals for Partnership with the Public*, which she produced as a resource for a symposium entitled 'Letter sharing has it all', held in London in March 2002. Copies of the bibliography are obtainable from www.4Ps.org.uk.

References

1   Baldry M, Cheal C, Fisher B *et al.* (1986) Giving patients their own records in general practice: experience of patients and staff. *BMJ.* **292**: 595–9.

2   Electronic Patient Record: a report on this initiative can be found at the 'Office of the e-Envoy' Cabinet Office website; www.e-envoy.gov.uk/oee/oee.nsf/sections/index/$file/index.htm

3   Stevens MM (1992) 'Shuttle Sheet': a patient-held medical record for paediatric oncology families. *Med Paediatr Oncol.* **20**: 330–35.

4   Drury M, Yudkin P, Harcourt J *et al.* (2000) Patients with cancer holding their own records: a randomised controlled trial. *Br J Gen Pract.* **50**: 105–10.

5   Jones R, McConville J, Mason D *et al.* (1999) Attitudes towards, and utility of, an integrated medical–dental patient-held record in primary care. *Br J Gen Pract.* **49**: 368–73.

6   Scott JT, Entwhistle VA, Sowdon AJ *et al.* (2001) Recordings or summaries of consultations for people with cancer (Cochrane Review). In: *The Cochrane Library. Issue 3.* Update Software, Oxford.

7   Hamilton W, Round A and Sharp D (1999) Effect on hospital attendance rates of giving patients a copy of their referral letter: randomised controlled trial. *BMJ.* **318**: 392–4.

8   Jelley D and van Zwanenberg T (2000) Copying general practitioner referral letters to patients: a study of patients' views. *Br J Gen Pract.* **50**: 657–8.

9   Jelley D, van Zwanenberg T and Scott D (2003) Copying letters to patients – the implications for policy implementation. *Prim Health Care Res Dev.* In press.

10   Department of Health (2000) *The NHS Plan for England and Wales.* The Stationery Office, London.

11   Guadagnoli E and Ward P (1998) Patient participation in decision making. *Soc Sci Med.* **47**: 329–39.

12   Department of Health (1999) *Patient and Public Involvement in the New NHS;* www.doh.gov.uk/coinh.htm

13   Duman M and Farrell C (2000) *Practicalities of Producing Patient Information: the POPPI guide.* The King's Fund, London.

14   Jadad A (1999) Promoting partnerships – challenges for the Internet Age. *BMJ.* **319**: 761–4.

15   Pal B (1999) Email contact between doctor and patient. *BMJ.* **318**: 1428.

16   Plain English Campaign (2001) *How to Write Medical Information in Plain English.* Plain English Campaign, High Peak. www.plainenglish.co.uk

17   White M and Epston D (1989) *Literate Means to Therapeutic Ends.* Dulwich Centre Publications, Adelaide.

18   O'Connor A *et al.* (1999) Decision aids for patients facing health treatment or screening decisions: systematic review. *BMJ.* **319**: 731–4.

19   Coulter A, Entwistle V and Gilbert D (1999) Sharing decisions with patients: is the information good enough? *BMJ.* **318**: 318–22.

20   Edwards A and Elwyn G (2001) Understanding risk and lessons for clinical risk communication about treatment preferences. *Qual Health Care.* **10**: 9–13.

21   Hugman R (1991) *Power in Caring Professions.* Macmillan, Basingstoke.

22   Øvretveit J (1993) *Co-ordinating Community Care: multidisciplinary teams and care management*. Open University Press, Buckingham.

23   Stevenson O and Parsloe P (1993) *Community Care and Empowerment*. Joseph Rowntree Foundation, York.

24   Department of Health (2000) *The Health and Social Care Bill*. The Stationery Office, London.

25   Dale N (1996) *Working with Families of Children with Special Needs: partnership and practice*. Routledge, London.

26   Spencer J, Blackmore D, Heard S *et al.* (2000) Patient-oriented learning: a review of the role of the patient in the education of medical students. *Med Educ.* **34**: 851–6.

27   DAFNE Study Group (2002) Training in flexible, intensive insulin management to enable dietary freedom in people with type 1 diabetes: dose adjustment for normal eating (DAFNE) randomised controlled trial. *BMJ.* **325**: 746.

28   Chambers R (2001) *Involving Patients and the Public: how to do it better*. Radcliffe Medical Press, Oxford.

CHAPTER 13

People and places

Liz Haggard

This chapter explores how buildings can contribute to increasing the level of trust in the healthcare system.

Introduction

Children learn about which types of people to trust and which to treat with suspicion. They also learn about places – those to avoid, which are dangerous and dirty, and those which are clean, nice, attractive and safe.

Indeed, most aspects of trust and distrust are learned in childhood. Good judgement – about whom and what to trust – is an important advantage for navigating through life. Where daily routine and a restricted geographical world limit the number of encounters with novel situations, people learn to trust the familiar. Those who attend one surgery and one hospital throughout their lifetime come to trust that familiar healthcare environment. Today's geographically mobile population will experience a number of different healthcare environments and, with increasing specialisation, will attend a range of different hospitals. If such places risk being perceived as untrustworthy because they are unfamiliar, can we build trust in other ways? And does it matter if we do not do so?

This chapter seeks to look at the role which health service buildings can play in making patients feel more trust – or distrust – in healthcare services.

Healthcare buildings and the social map

Healthcare buildings occupy a special place on the social and cultural map. Inevitably, expectations arise about how doctors' surgeries, hospitals and nursing homes should look and function. Hospitals were originally founded and run by religious and voluntary institutions, and to some degree they retain aspects of the 'sacred'. Thus when hospitals began to introduce commercial shops, many people felt uncomfortable about mixing secular commerce with sacred healing. Healthcare buildings must also serve the whole population, and there will be a range of expectations about how a hospital or a doctor's surgery should look. Martin Amis, describing the Chelsea and Westminster Hospital, wrote about the entrance hall – much admired by architects and designers, but so unlike his idea of a hospital. He was visiting his dying father at the time. No doubt he would have preferred something more 'hospital-like'.

However, most of the users of health services are older people, whose expectations were shaped 40 or 50 years ago through their experience of hospitals with imposing entrances, shining brass, polished linoleum floors and a wood-panelled hall. Younger patients (the older people of the future) will expect something more like the modern public and commercial buildings of today.

Different hospital users feel comfortable in different surroundings. A day hospital for older people ought to look and feel different from a day hospital where most of the patients are young, though shared public areas need to be able to reassure everyone.

Local communities display passionate attachments to their hospital buildings, conscious both of their underlying 'sacredness' and of their familiarity. Such familiarity is a key component of trust, and helps to explain the numerous examples of local campaigns to save much-loved buildings, which are often more than 100 years old.

Nineteenth-century buildings and twenty-first-century healthcare

It is hard to deliver twenty-first century healthcare in nineteenth-century buildings. The familiarity of the old building may lead to misplaced trust – looking and feeling trustworthy is not the only consideration. Inevitably, as healthcare has become both more complex and more dependent on technology, the requirements placed on buildings have also increased. The public rightly expects such complexity to be well managed – buildings must balance technical issues with patient-trustworthy design.

For example, technical requirements make it difficult to produce an up-to-date operating theatre which allows the patient to feel instantly at ease (although, for watchers of TV hospital dramas, it may at least look familiar!).

However, within the limits of technical requirements it is possible to design an environment which increases trust by:

• showing patients that someone has thought about their expectations
• trying to make the environment attractive
• minimising the visibility of elements that are likely to be alarming.

There are many examples of maternity suites where mothers give birth in technically well-equipped rooms which are also attractive and reassuring. Children's wards and operating theatres also look radically different, with staff, parents and children working together. Hospitals now realise that patients lying on trolleys or in bed have only the ceiling to look at for much of the time. There are major gains in moving from a plain white ceiling with fluorescent lighting (plus a dead fly or two) to an attractively painted ceiling (and not a dead fly in sight).

Certain buildings progressively inhibit the capacity for patients and staff to develop trust. Patients withhold the trust they would like to feel, and rationalise their unease ('It's a bit shabby, but the doctors and nurses are lovely'). Staff feel less supported ('We're doing our best in difficult circumstances'). How important it is then to modify such a building in order to make patients and staff feel well cared for and understood. They are then more likely to trust both the organisation and each other.

Clean, clean, clean

The most reassuring characteristic for patients is cleanliness. This means cleanliness that they can see and smell – a building may be technically clean but look scruffy, and it can of course look clean but be technically dirty. Patients are the only relevant judges of the former, and expert staff of the latter, but both are important. Achieving and maintaining patient-visible and technically measurable cleanness is difficult. It requires endless maintenance and attention to detail in an area of work which is usually seen as low status, and where pay and conditions are poor. It also requires quality materials which will remain in good condition under the heavy wear and tear of health service use. Saving money by laying down poor-quality carpet or omitting skirting boards will ensure that, soon enough, patients will see scruffy carpet and scuffed walls, and cleaning staff will feel that their task is hopeless.

It seems astonishing that the high value which patients place on cleanliness has had to be rediscovered at national level, and that we needed to have a Clean Hospitals Plan to remind us that:

> Patients expect certain things of the NHS. They expect high-quality care in hospitals that are clean, tidy and welcoming. They do not expect dirty wards, smelly toilets, shabby surroundings or poor food.[1]

For older generations of staff and patients, the NHS obsession with cleanliness was a given, and it took some years of shrinking budgets and the requirement to privatise cleaning services for patients' concerns to be heard and action taken. The current focus on cleanliness, reflected in the work of the Patient Environment Action Teams (PEATs) and of the Commission for Health Improvement (CHI) inspections of hospitals and surgeries, has moved all aspects of cleanliness up the agenda.

People × buildings = complexity

The multiplicity of sensations and the subliminal awareness which make us feel that a building is trustworthy are complex. Although cleanness is a basic requirement, it will not in itself deliver trust. The positive impact of the cleanest and most attractive surgery will be wiped out by a tactless or rude receptionist or an hour-long wait to see the doctor. Reflecting on other services, such as those provided by a café, exposes the attention to detail that is required in order to build trust – how things to do with the building and things to do with people interact (*see* Box 13.1).

Box 13.1   They're doing their best at the new local café, but …

It's a brand new building, very smart looking	It was very hard to find because they hadn't thought about signposting and it didn't look like a café
The décor in the dining room is wonderful and it looks really clean and fresh	The toilets were filthy and there was no toilet paper

The staff were really great – friendly and professional	The staff seemed great, but when I went back next week the staff were all different – I don't like that
It's in a lovely country park outside town	There was nowhere to park and the bus service is lousy and it's miles from anywhere
It's very busy – lots of people, not a vacant table	It was very noisy and there were lots of smokers
The food looked lovely and the china was very elegant	The food took ages to come and we were all ill next day
It was all very modern and colourful	The décor was fine for the young people, but I like something more restful

Buildings blindness

People who work in the health services find it difficult to see their buildings from the perspective of a new or anxious patient. Therefore the easiest way of getting it right is to 'rent a patient' – ask two or three people to visit as if they were first-time patients. Ask them how the building strikes them. Then make changes, and ask them back again. If they do not mention that it feels and looks clean, you have a problem with a core requirement, and you need to take urgent action.

However, patients are not expert designers. They will not know what is needed to make buildings look and feel trustworthy. Expert designers should advise on colour, texture, lighting, materials, patterns and all of the complex factors which can make a building a delight – they also need to have additional specialist know-ledge about health service buildings and their specific requirements. The cost of such design expertise (compared with the cost of the building, furnishing or deco-rating work in the life of the building) is minimal. The cost of not using design expertise is obvious in far too many of our health services buildings.

The halo of shabbiness

For some people the shabbiness of NHS premises came to have a counter-intuitive value. It is as if they said:

> Look at this, so shabby and uncomfortable. It is clearly not a profit-making business but something different, which values treatment and care more than pretty curtains or shining floors. Although the place is grubby, the staff will be angels with hearts of gold and healing hands, working against insuperable odds.

Shabbiness came to signal trustworthy services – a reminder of the shared values (and privations) of the war years, the world of the creation of the NHS. Today shabbiness is no longer a trait to be forgiven, but a confirmation that all may not be well.

How to make buildings feel untrustworthy

Information about how buildings may increase trust is available from a number of sources.[2,3] Some of this information is based on research.[4] It is clear that patients prefer buildings which are visually attractive, with reception desks designed to invite patients to ask for help. In general, they dislike loud or constant noise and unpleasant smells, they appreciate privacy (as well as cleanliness) in the toilet and bathroom, and they prefer hot and attractively presented food, curtains which are not falling off the curtain rail, colour schemes which go beyond magnolia, clear signposting, and furniture which is both comfortable and attractive!

Guidance is also available on technical aspects. NHS buildings have to conform to the usual regulations with regard to access, fire escapes and toilet facilities, as well as to those regulations which are specific to hospitals and nursing homes. However, such regulations may not address issues of how to increase trustworthiness. Box 13.2 highlights ways of reducing such trust.

Box 13.2   Easy and effective ways of creating unease and lack of trust

- Poor-quality signposting outside the hospital so that patient and visitors feel confused and uncertain even before they enter the building
- A variety of entrances to the hospital building which are not designed to be highly visible, so that patients do not know which is the right entrance
- A complicated map of the site which most people find difficult to follow
- A water feature such as a pond with paper bags floating in it
- A carpet of cigarette butts leading to the main entrance
- A few items of equipment at the entrance (broken wheelchairs of zimmer-frames are ideal)
- An overflowing rubbish bin
- Weeds, crisp packets and some dead plants in the flower-beds

---

By contrast, attractive environments enhance care. One study in the USA showed that length of stay was reduced if patients could see natural scenes from a window, or even a good-quality picture of a nature scene.[5] Recent research in the UK has confirmed what common sense tells us – that good design can reduce length of stay and increase confidence among staff.[6]

Help with healing buildings

NHS Estates has been through as many changes as the rest of the NHS, and the use of Private Finance Initiative (PFI) funding for big capital projects is a major change in the way in which public sector buildings are funded and maintained. It is too early to say whether the higher cost of raising capital in this way will speed up the replacement of the worst buildings and improve quality and suitability in the longer term. New hospitals are now designed by staff whose experience is increasingly in the commercial non-health sector, taking advice from the health service. This has positive and negative effects – positive learning from successes in other public contexts (e.g. hotels, department stores and office buildings), but negative effects where designs fail to understand how hospitals work.

NHS Estates leads on the AEDET project (Achieving Excellence – Design Evaluation Toolkit)[7] and offers Web-based examples of designs for hospitals and surgeries (with solutions to common health service building problems).[8] An NHS Research Group has been established, building on the work of long-established groups such as the Medical Architecture Research Group (MARU). NHS Estates has also set up a network of Design Champions to promote good design, and it recently commissioned a series of well-illustrated books on ways of making health services buildings more attractive, the first being *The Art of Good Health: using the visual arts in healthcare*. A practical handbook on how to set up an arts programme is also available.[9] Other books in the series will look at specific topics, such as reception areas. The books illustrate good ideas and design solutions, summarise research findings and provide useful contact addresses.

Building for the future

A good building can create a sense of therapeutic optimism for staff and patients alike, dispelling previous feelings of struggle and strain. The latest NHS *Priorities and Planning Framework 2003–2006* states that with regard to 'physical facilities' the objective is:

> To create a clean, comfortable, well-maintained physical environment, which is fit to deliver modern, convenient care. This includes delivering sufficient physical capacity in the right place to implement the NHS's key priorities, increasing diversity of provision through use of non-NHS providers where appropriate, and ensuring that physical facilities are modernised in line with the vision set out in the NHS Plan.

Thus there are to be 29 new hospitals by June 2005, and there is a national target of 3000 GP premises to be refurbished or replaced by the end of 2004, 500 one-stop primary care centres, and new Diagnostic and Treatment Centres, with at least 40% of the 'total value of the NHS estate to be less than 15 years old by 2010'. There appears to be a real desire to give NHS staff and patients buildings designed for twenty-first-century healthcare.

The Wanless Report explores the kind of health service that is needed to meet future patient expectations and become a 'responsive world-class service'. It is a good source of information about patient views and priorities.[10] The report comments on the need to improve and modernise hospital buildings, in the light of a massive maintenance backlog which Wanless quotes as being in excess of £3 billion.

NHS Estates assumes an asset life for buildings of 60 years, so what is built today must cater for the needs of contemporary 20-year-olds when they become octogenarians. Already people would like an attractive single room, meals and snacks to order, and en-suite facilities when they go into hospital. In technical terms this is possible, and financially it may well be affordable because of the resulting reduction in cross-infection and intensive cleaning. However, we have to build for it now (the move from Nightingale wards to bays of six patients took years, and we still have Nightingale wards today).

The family doctor surgery

Although hospitals have a powerful symbolic importance for the cultural map of cities and communities, most health service experience is in general practice. Traditionally, the surgery was a local building, often the doctor's own house, and it changed little over the years.

Compared with a visit to hospital, general practice should feel more familiar, less impersonal and more predictable. Over the last 20 years the numbers of staff, the way in which they work and the range of services that they offer have increased dramatically. Yet all too often the surgery buildings have not changed a great deal. One of the reasons for this lack of change is the system which funds general practice and surgery buildings. GPs may 'own' their premises, but to a large extent these buildings are paid for – albeit in a labyrinthine way – by the NHS.

A recent Audit Commission report[11] found that many surgeries did not meet even basic standards (e.g. 30% were found to have inadequate hand-washing facilities). The new primary care trusts (PCTs) will be expected to clarify standards, and CHI inspection visits aim to highlight problems. Upgrading GP surgeries is complex, especially in major cities where space is limited and land values are high. Finding space to park and providing access and facilities for disabled people often prove difficult because of building constraints. The NHS usually contributes to the cost of surgery improvement, but the practice partnership will also have to raise money, and it may be unwilling or unable to do this. Despite these difficulties, many practices have modernised their surgery premises, and there are some good illustrated examples on the NHS Estates primary care website.[12]

The introduction to the website sets out the direction that the Government wishes to pursue, quoting from the NHS Plan:

> Many GPs will be working in teams from modern multi-purpose premises alongside nurses, pharmacists, dentists, therapists, opticians, midwives and social care staff. Nurses will have new opportunities, and some GPs will tend to specialise in treating different conditions. The consulting-room will become the place where appointments for out-patients and operations are booked, test results received and more diagnosis carried out using video and tele-links to hospital specialists. An increasing number of consultants will take outpatient sessions in local primary care centres.[12]

Such ambitions are not new. The NHS has a history of building health centres to accommodate GPs, nurses and other community-based clinicians, with mixed results. However, many GPs prefer the 'independence' of owning and managing their own premises. GPs who moved into health centres often found the NHS slow to respond to requests for alterations, repairs and improvements. Placing GPs with other community staff in the same premises did not always lead to better communication or mutual trust. Where two or three GP practices shared the same health centre there were often tensions. Each practice would retain its own working arrangements, highlighting the fact that co-operation and synergy cannot be imposed by co-location – although co-location, and a wider range of services offered, may be more convenient for patients.

Current policy continues to encourage GPs to modernise their premises, especially through the PFI. Primary care trusts are responsible for planning and prioritising improvements. The dilemma remains whether to give priority to those who run efficient, popular practices in good premises, who wish to expand further, or to those whose buildings and services need to be brought up to modern standards. The inverse-care law applies equally to premises – the neediest populations tend to have the poorest premises – but complex issues of how to share out scarce resources remain.

One other initiative is the Local Improvement Finance Trust (LIFT). This recognises that individual surgeries and NHS clinics are too small to interest private investors and builders, but that by bringing together a number of buildings in a geographical area the size of a PCT, there may be a large enough project to attract private finance investment.[13]

In assessing how best to provide high-quality accessible, and attractive healthcare services, it is also necessary to note the following.

- Buildings are often in the wrong place – they are where the population used to be, not where it is now.
- The best-looking buildings are within the better-off communities.
- There are too many buildings, which for much of the time are not in full use.
- There is duplication of facilities.
- Some buildings are so ugly that they will never be attractive to either staff or patients.
- None of the buildings have adequate car parking facilities.

LIFT managers are now being appointed by primary care trusts to tackle these issues. Yet the agenda remains vast. The Audit Commission report already cited[11] states that one in ten of all general practices (increasing to one in three in London) fails to meet basic standards (e.g. adequate heating in waiting-rooms, clean facilities in good repair, adequate toilet and washing facilities, and proper fire escapes).

Changing the light bulb can make a big difference: the 'Modern Matrons' initiative

Most NHS staff can tell stories of how long it took to get the new shelf, the notice board, the grab rail, or the replacement for the torn curtain or the broken blind. Petty rules and demarcation disputes block progress and sensible solutions. One response to this has been the creation of the 'Modern Matron'. Modern Matrons take responsibility for practical matters. Each has a personal budget of £5000 to improve life on the ward, although guidelines on how to spend this are somewhat complicated.[14]

Giving Modern Matrons money to spend has an immediate appeal, but could it also be unwise? For surely if we really cared about the quality of the patient environment, we would ask those with real expertise in design issues. Design expertise, like nursing expertise, has to be studied and practised. The King's Fund, which has an honourable track record of interest in designing patient-friendly health service buildings, recognises this and has established an initiative which gives nurses access to design expertise, understanding about how to make a positive difference, and time to think through their ideas.

Enhancing the healing environment

This scheme, which was launched in January 2001,[15] has already given grants of £35 000 to each of 33 London hospitals to undertake environmental improvements in patient areas. Projects range from refurbishment to the introduction of artworks and landscaping. Examples have included replacing the harsh strip-lighting of an Accident and Emergency department with softer lighting, thereby creating a more homely atmosphere.

Lighting is a good example of the need for both design and clinical expertise. Knowing the type and intensity of light which will be aesthetically pleasing in particular settings requires design knowledge, skills and experience. Clinical expertise points out which areas need high-intensity full-spectrum lighting.

Choosing colours, patterns, textures and flooring which are technically acceptable, easy to maintain and aesthetically pleasing to the majority of people is more complex. Deciding on pictures, murals or music may prove more complicated still. For example, when Charles Saatchi donated modern art pieces to the Chelsea and Westminster Hospital, not all of them were accepted (a sequence involving chickens with severed heads was not regarded as appropriate for display in a hospital!). However, charities such as Paintings in Hospital can give advice on such matters.

- People learn to trust both individuals and environments.
- Buildings engender strong emotions.
- Cleanliness is now back on the agenda.
- Technical needs must be balanced by patient-friendly design.
- Good design increases patient and staff satisfaction and leads to better outcomes for all.
- A series of new initiatives is helping to enhance the therapeutic environment.

References

1   For more details about the Clean Hospitals plan, see http://www.clean hospitals.com/home/index.asp

2   Hosking S and Haggard L (1999) *Healing the Hospital Environment: design, management and maintenance of healthcare premises.* SPON Press, London.

3   The NHS Estates Design Portfolio illustrates building design solutions that respond to common challenges faced by the NHS. The schemes range from acute hospitals to primary care practices. All buildings have been included on the basis of their own merit and substantiated by the opinion of patients, staff and visitors; www.nhsdesignportfolio.nhsestates.gov.uk

4   NHS Estates produce a CD-ROM which summarises a number of their research studies and gives details of other research. Details are available at http://www.nhsestates.gov.uk/training_r_and_d/index.asp

5   Ulrich RS (1997) Theory of supportive design for healthcare environments. *J Healthcare Design.* **9**: 3–7.

6   Purvis A (2001) Health buildings design. *Guardian Health.* **5 July**.

7   AEDET (Achieving Excellence – Design Evaluation Toolkit) www.nhsestates. gov.uk/download/AEDET

8   www.nhsestates.gov.uk/patient_environment

9   NHS Estates (2002) *The Art of Good Health: using the visual arts in healthcare.* NHS Estates, London.

10   Wanless D (2002) *Securing Our Future Health: taking a long-term view. The final report;* www.hm-treasury.gov.uk/Consultations_and_Legislation/wanless/consult_wanless_final.cfm

11   Audit Commission (2002) *The Performance of the NHS in England: developing an independent commentary;* www.audit-commission.gov.uk

12   www.nhsestates.gov.uk/primary_care/index.asp

13   www.nhsestates.gov.uk/primary_care/index.asp

14   www.purchasingcard.nhs.uk

15   Contact the King's Fund, 11–13 Cavendish Square, London W1M 0AN. Tel: 020 7307 2400. Email: libweb@kingsfund.org.uk. Web: www.kingsfund. org.uk

CHAPTER 14

Learning from business

Robin McKenzie

In country banking, intricate and often nationwide webs of marriage, especially among Quakers, created a network of trust, which spanned commercial, financial and industrial interests.[1]

> This chapter describes changes in western business over the last 20 years. It suggests that a culture based on 'control' is giving way to a new emphasis on trust-based human relationships, which is affecting all areas of company activity.

Introduction

Is business just 'business', making profit through a set of tasks and objectives? Or is business a set of relationships? We might be inclined to the former view, but consider the (albeit fictional) *Postman Pat* (distribution), *Bob the Builder* (construction) or *The Archers* (agricultural business), where business tasks are only a vehicle to enable personal relationships to be enacted, grow and develop. This chapter will suggest that relationships have more importance in business than people generally realise.

We do not naturally expect the world of business to supply us with models of good human relating. Often we experience business relationships in assertive or even aggressive contexts. We tolerate business because it provides the products and services that we need, but we secretly despise its greed and self-interest. The accounting scandals of Enron and Worldcom confirm our prejudices. In the UK, the problems of the railways continue to make headlines, whether due to severe delays or tragic accidents. Do we trust private companies not to take shortcuts with safety? Looking further back, the UK has had its own financial scandals, notably the money-laundering activities of the Bank of Commerce and Credit International (BCCI), and Robert Maxwell's bullying and stealing from his company's pension fund. So it may seem strange to look to business for examples of trusting behaviour.

Yet the last 20 years have seen a sea change in many industries. Where previously there was distance and control, now there are partnerships and trusting relationships. Of course, trust depends in part on the attitudes, values and beliefs of individuals – but trust exists between people. Hence, for trust to flourish, the individual must become part of a larger network whose activities and structures are oriented towards furthering trusting behaviours. This applies both within organisations and between organisations. Moreover, these changes in patterns of relating in business have had a significant impact on the quality of services provided to customers. Business no longer stands apart from those whom it seeks to serve.

Two approaches to relationships in business: control or relate

We can envisage two very different patterns of relating in business. The first can be 'control-based relating'. According to this model, business is all about the control of people, materials and processes in order to satisfy business objectives. Power is held centrally and at the top of the company. This is the view of business that is held by the general public.

The second type of business relating we can term 'relational relating'. Here the people who make up the business are emphasised. Business is seen as a vehicle for individuals and groups to pursue creative and purposeful lives. This is the view of popular drama.

In so far as real business has an interest in relationships, these are of course the kind of relationships that are concerned with the furtherance of business activity, not the fostering of the private and personal relationships beloved of the dramatist. However, over the last ten years, relationships in business have moved into the centre of the picture, with business experiencing a widespread shift from control-based relating to relational relating.

This chapter provides some background information about how businesses came to be 'control-based'. It explains how a (somewhat caricatured) control-based business operates. It then shows how, particularly in response to the impact of Japanese competition, business began to adopt a very different culture of relating. The way in which a contemporary, 'relationally rich' business conducts itself is discussed. Finally, some suggestions for applications to the field of medicine and healthcare are given.

How control-based businesses came into being

Developed control-based business, as seen clearly in the 1960s and 1970s, is based on a quasi-scientific view of business activity allied to particular structures of economics and law which distance people from one another.

Adam Smith, the founder of modern economics, conceived of the economy as being composed of individual, autonomous companies, each in competition with the others. Within a company, work ought to be broken down into its constituent parts and the efficiency of each part maximised. Smith is well known for his example of the pin factory, where 10 men are needed to perform the 10 separate operations involved in making a pin.[2]

Towards the end of the nineteenth century, a manager in an American steel company believed that he could motivate his workforce by giving more pay to those who worked harder. Frederick Taylor invented the first modern incentive system for production operators, published in 1911.[3] Such 'Scientific Management' was based on an objective understanding of the content of the tasks that individuals undertake. Workers were conceived of mechanistically, and motivation of people was regarded as straightforward – more pay for more work.

Both Smith's and Taylor's theories depend on an understanding of human society that is drawn from the natural sciences.[4] For Adam Smith, economics and moral reasoning were both based on natural laws.[5] Human society was pictured as a great machine, one part of which was business. Research and experimentation on such a 'machine' were thus legitimate, and arguably this led to the exploitation of workers within the growing industries of Victorian Britain. The 'machine' understanding of business served to distance the privileged few (owners and bosses) from the disadvantaged many (employees and workers).

This distancing was reinforced by two other important steps, namely the creation of limited liability joint stock legislation, and the introduction of mass production.

Nineteenth-century legislation enabling the creation of limited liability joint stock companies[1,6] meant that, should a company fail, any investor would be liable only for the amount originally invested, rather than for any larger debt now owed. This legislation provided the means for forming the first large industrial organisations – the railway companies. Joint stock limited liability allowed the investor to distance himself from his company while still sharing in its ownership.

In 1913, Henry Ford invented 'mass production' using the moving conveyor built at his Highland Park factory in Detroit.[7] Although many of the individual practices of mass production (such as the division of labour into its smallest parts) already existed, it was Ford who put the whole set of practices together. A moving assembly line brought work to the worker, reduced walking time, and set the pace of the work to be done. The production process gained a new level of transparent, controlled efficiency. Cars were produced at unprecedentedly low cost.

Thus economics derived from Adam Smith, legal structures which distanced owners from their investments, motivational theories based on 'scientific management', and production-line manufacturing techniques together combined to foster a 'machine-like' view of the human worker, in which 'trust' and 'human relationships' easily disappeared from view.

Control as the primary relationship

Let us now consider what a control-based company looks and feels like. In this (somewhat caricatured) company, direction comes from the top and is cascaded down. I shall suggest what this means for six key aspects of business activity, namely finance, customers, internal (production) processes, suppliers, personnel and innovation.

Finance

In a control-based company, financial assessment is the main (or even only) way of assessing performance. The 'numbers' derived from accounting practices are seen to be objective and measurable. These numbers, which include production figures, costing, overheads and pricing, are combined and recombined to give an assessment of the company and its position in the market. Notice that in the USA there is an especially high dependence on numbers, with publicly quoted companies required to report quarterly (compared with a biannual requirement in the UK). In this type of company and culture, it is the supposedly 'hard' financial information which is trusted.

Customers

In its dealings with customers, the control-based company concentrates on the immediate sale. For this type of company, after-sales concerns, especially customer complaints, are seen as a nuisance. Long-term customer retention and loyalty is a useful by-product, but not the main focus. Customers are not trusted – they are viewed as tools for the benefit of the company.

Internal (production) process

Responsibility for the production processes within a control-based company lies with departments. Each department is fully responsible for its own set of processes and procedures, and its managers are measured and rewarded against specified measurable targets. This is not a 'one-off' event but a year-on-year process, where performance is required to increase steadily. Departments are separate from one another and have only limited and formal contact with each other.

Although the manager of the department may have some limited input into the targets to be achieved, in a control-based company these are usually set by some higher authority and imposed downwards. The 'numbers' are trusted more than the opinions of departmental managers.

Suppliers

Suppliers are dealt with by a distant, arm's-length approach. They must provide quotations and deliver goods against detailed sets of requirements given by the company. Each supplier must deliver when the company wants, however disruptive this might prove to the supplier. The only financial information that is exchanged between the company and the supplier is the price charged for the product or service. No underlying costing information (e.g. such as would provide evidence as to whether or not the supplier is able to make a profit) is exchanged. The relationship is set out in a detailed contract, with many clauses and subclauses, so that the company can obtain legal redress from the supplier if things go wrong. The company does not trust the supplier. It also has the ability to change supplier frequently, as contracts for supply only last for one year.

As a consequence of the company not trusting its supplier to deal responsibly with subcontractors, it must deal with every potential supplier itself. For example, in the case of a car manufacturer, the company might have to deal with several thousand individual suppliers.

Personnel

The attitude of a control-based company to its employees is conflictual and paradoxical. Some employees are regarded as potential 'stars' and are given opportunities to develop and progress through the company. By contrast, the main bulk of employees, including operators and technicians, are expected to arrive in the company with limited competency, and training is only directed at these employees in the required, rather narrow, competencies of their duties.

In this way, the company divides its employees into two groups – the minority whom it will trust, train and promote, and the majority whom it does not trust and whom it will ignore.

Innovation

No market, business or company can stay the same and survive. It must discover, develop and introduce new ideas and products. In a control-based company, where only a limited handful of employees are trusted, innovation must come through this limited source. Even when an idea is generated externally, it has to come from a reputable outside source, and then through a 'gatekeeper' who is one of these trusted employees. In other words, there is only a limited and inflexible set of procedures for the introduction and exploitation of innovation.

Trust in business today: relational relationship rediscovered

Control-based approaches were prevalent in western businesses up until about 20 years ago. So, we might ask, why the change? What made us come to our senses and gave us a new perception of people's worth? The answer is surprisingly simple, and can be summed up in one word – the Japanese. In the 1970s, a range of products, especially cars, cameras and electronic goods, started to appear in western countries at low prices, with superior quality and immediate availability. The result was devastating. For example, the British motorcycle industry – the largest such manufacturer in the world in the 1950s – was decimated, and the British car industry was only kept afloat during the 1970s by large Government subsidies.

The arrival of the Japanese

The Japanese seemed to be doing the impossible – selling quality products at low prices. Naturally there were suspicions of unfair trade. The Japanese were accused of selling products at below their manufacturing cost. In reality, western business productivity was considerably lower than that of the Japanese. Even in 1989, following some considerable catching up, it still took twice as long on average to produce a car in Europe as in Japan.[7]

A proper understanding of why the Japanese were successful emerged only gradually. Their productivity was attributed at first to a variety of supposedly miraculous production techniques. However, it eventually became clear that there was one fundamental difference between western and Japanese business, and this was the attitude of the Japanese to relationships. For the Japanese, relationships – all relationships – were important. Relationships were not just about feelings or words, but were expressed in a set of practices that produced quantifiable business benefits. Such benefits included a reduction in the time and cost of bringing a new product to the market, a quantum change in attitude to quality, a sharing of information and personnel, and the subcontracting of whole sub-assemblies (e.g. headlight assemblies and sunroof assemblies in car production) to specialist subcontractors.

Discovering the new or recovering the old?

Although 'the Japanese way' seemed radical, the valuing of relationships is by no means a new concept or a new way of doing business. Before the legal development of 'limited liability' in the nineteenth century, business relationships were essentially personal relationships. Where investors were personally liable for company losses (as still applies to the Names of Lloyd's of London), and had little recourse should another party renege on part of the deal, it was vital to know and trust the people with whom one did business. Business was conducted within a network of people and relationships, characterised by trust, transparency, reputation and audit, not by directing command or hierarchical control. A prime example of this network of personal relationships is that established by the Quaker families in the business life of nineteenth-century Britain. Their success was due in part to formal and informal means of meeting and auditing each other, as well as to their national structures, in which personal contacts and recommendations could take place.

The relationally-based company

Let us now consider what the 'relational' company looks like. We shall take the same areas of business life that we looked at with the control-based company. However, the order will be different, as befits a different set of priorities.

Innovation

It is in the area of design and innovation that the greatest benefits of a relationally based company are generated. Traditionally, all design work was done sequentially. Only when one stage of the design work was completed was it passed on (*see* Figure 14.1a). The advantage of this method was that difficulties within any one stage were dealt with there and then.

However, good design is often the result of holding together different, often competing design criteria. For example, there is a trade-off between toughness and flexibility, the cost of buying in components rather than producing them internally, the requirement for higher-quality products for a specified market against the additional cost, and so on. The sequential model struggles with these subtleties.

If there is communication between different departments and stages in the design project, not only might the project be completed in a fraction of the time, but also many potential problems might be overcome on the way. This second type of design is called *simultaneous design* or *concurrent engineering* (*see* Figure 14.1b).

Changing from sequential to concurrent design can result – and indeed has resulted – in some startling savings in lead times for bringing products to market. It requires a much higher level of trust and co-operation between departments than would be expected or needed in a control-based company.

(a)

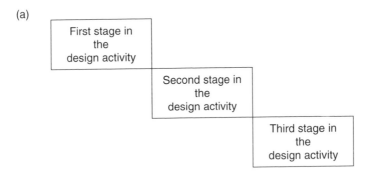

(b)

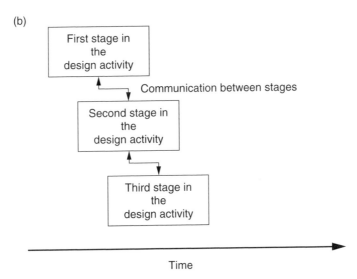

Time

Figure 14.1   Design methods. (a) Sequential design. (b) Simultaneous design or concurrent engineering. *Source*: Slack *et al.*[8]

Personnel

A relationally based company treats everyone as important, not just the privileged few. The Japanese expressed this in their policy of retaining all workers once they were employed (although the current and enduring difficulties within the Japanese economy have significantly eroded this commitment). Engaging with all employees means training and support for all (*see also* Box 14.1).[9]

Box 14.1   National cultures and social capital

Francis Fukuyama, the American management scholar, argues that the quality of business relationships is a reflection of the form of relationships in wider national culture.[10] Fukuyama argues that the key factor in national culture is the encouragement it gives to individuals to associate outside their kinship group.

Most businesses start as family concerns. If they cannot easily bring in non-family members as the business grows, then the limiting size of the business is the size of the family. Fukuyama calls this ability to associate *social capital*. Japan, the USA and Germany have a high ability to associate, so have high social capital, whereas France and Korea have low social capital. The UK is somewhere in the middle.

Returning to the example of the Quakers, it is likely that the reason why they did not continue to be the force in business that they had been at the beginning of the twentieth century is that their only means of expansion was by employing senior managers from outside the sect. In time, therefore, the distinctiveness of the Quaker calling, with its associated benefits, was lost.

Interestingly, Fukuyama's analysis provides a set of criteria which put the advanced economies of the USA and Japan into the same group. Americans are normally viewed as individualistic and the Japanese as group-oriented, yet both are open to people who are not 'family'.

Customers

The relational business appreciates the importance of long-term relationships with customers. It knows that it costs much less to keep an established customer than to find the elusive new one.[11] The proliferation of loyalty-card schemes introduced by almost all of the main UK retailers illustrates the point well.

The change in the relationship between companies and their customers reflects an approach called *relationship marketing*. Table 14.1 compares the characteristics of relationship marketing with those of *transactional marketing* (the traditional approach taken to customers).

Internal (production) processes

The relationally based company trusts its workers and gives them significant responsibility for the quality of their work. For example, workers may be responsible, with local managers, for suggesting improvements to products or processes

Table 14.1   Characteristics of transactional and relationship marketing (*Source*: Payne[12])

Transactional (traditional) marketing	*Relationship marketing*
Focus on single sales	Focus on customer retention
Orientation to product features	Orientation to customer value
Short timescales	Long timescales
Little emphasis on customer service	Strong customer service emphasis
Limited customer commitment	High level of customer commitment
Moderate customer contact	High level of customer contact
Quality is primarily a concern for production	Quality is the concern of all

to reduce cost or improve quality. One formalised way of relating workers, tasks and the company occurs in what are known as *quality circles*,[8] where suggestions must be considered by management in a suitably short time. Another example concerns the Japanese-style car production line, where workers can stop the line if there is a quality problem.[8]

In the relational company, the boundary between the 'internal' and the 'external' is blurred. Traditionally, 'inside' the company were its employees, its land, its buildings and its production facilities. Now employees may be 'contracted in' from a supplier or customer, land and buildings may be leased, and production facilities may only be paid for when used. This is called a 'resource-based' approach, as opposed to the traditional 'asset-based' approach.[13] For example, some of today's low-cost airlines may now only pay for the use of engines when they are in service, and may subcontract engine maintenance to a third party. These airlines understand their business to be taking customers to where they want to go, not providing an infrastructure that enables them to do so.

Relationally based companies make the customer — not internal processes or politics — the focus of their activity. For example, whereas a company would once have been organised around keeping the production line going at all costs, now companies try to move products and information through the company in response to customer needs.

Suppliers

The relationally based company does not keep all of its many suppliers at arm's length, but develops close relationships with a few favoured suppliers. Other suppliers deal with the favoured suppliers rather than with the main company itself. This makes for considerable administrative savings in credit control and financial review. For example, one UK-based Japanese car manufacturer has just 200 suppliers.

Suppliers now also need to be considerably more flexible in their delivery of goods. Car manufacturers expect deliveries even of a single component several times per day ('just-in-time') to be used on the car manufacturer's production line. Increased trust in this system means that stock levels can be reduced, for in a production environment stock acts as protection against suppliers not delivering.[8] If the relationship with the supplier is good, there may be no need to maintain stock.

A potential disadvantage of the newly configured supply chain is that some suppliers who used to supply directly are now 'further away'. One way of avoiding this difficulty is to get a group of such suppliers to work together in so-called 'supplier associations'. Issues and difficulties can then be solved together, and in cases where the customer company is creating the difficulties, common problems can be addressed.[14]

Contractual trust describes the normal business transactional relationship. *Competence trust* occurs when the parties trust each other because of the particular knowledge that one or both of them may possess. *Goodwill trust* occurs if there is a mutual open agreement with each other (*see* Box 14.2).

These types of trust are necessarily hierarchical because it is difficult, for instance, to build goodwill trust on poor performance or competence. In addition, the three

---

Box 14.2   Sako's theory of trust

Mari Sako reached her understanding of trust through research on UK and Japanese business.[15] She came to the conclusion that there are three types of trust, which are built over time in any business relationship. First, there is *contractual trust*, which is built on by *competence trust*, which is in turn built on by *goodwill trust* (*see* Figure 14.2). These types of trust are related hierarchically.

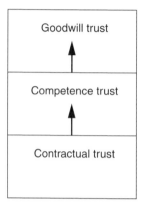

Figure 14.2   Hierarchical relationship between trust types. *Source*: Sako.[15]

types of trust can be placed on a continuum of trading relationships. At one end of the continuum is the *arm's-length contractual relation (ACR)*, where the contract is primary and the companies hold each other at a distance. At the other end of the continuum is the *obligation contractual relation (OCR)*, where the obligation overrides other considerations, at least in the short term.

The characteristics of the ACR are those outlined for control-based companies. Essentially all attitudes and behaviours between the companies are characterised by a lack of trust.

The OCR is characterised by high levels of trust and co-operation, by a commitment to trade over the long term, and by taking on of onerous obligations and requests (e.g. for just-in-time). Trust grows where there are mutual obligations towards and benefits from good quality and service, increasing orders and other non-price aspects of trading.

Sako's model is currently the simplest and clearest description of trust in business relationships.

Finance

In the relationally based company, although finance remains the final arbiter of company performance, financial reporting may be conducted and interpreted differently and set alongside the quality of relationships with suppliers and customers. One such approach is called the *balanced scorecard*, where company performance is

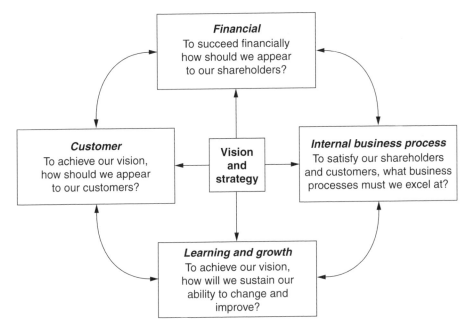

Figure 14.3   Balanced Scorecard. *Source*: Kaplan and Norton (adapted).[16]

assessed by a combination of financial data and information about customer relations, the success of internal business processes, and a score for innovation (*see* Figure 14.3).[16]

Conclusion: some suggestions for medicine and healthcare

This rediscovered approach to 'relational relationships' can provide successful examples of best practice which, in a modified form, could be applied to medicine and healthcare organisations.

Some possible implications of this business analysis are listed below.

- Input into innovation should be open to all healthcare workers, not just to healthcare managers or powerful interest groups such as the pharmaceutical suppliers.
- It is important to ask who are the gatekeepers of information. Should doctors be responsible for all decisions?
- Patients should be the genuine focus for healthcare. The organisational processes within medical care should be directed towards the patient, and not arranged for the convenience of medical professionals. Queues are like stock for business – they provide a comfort buffer for the organisation.
- Primary care and hospital medicine should be organised as one seamless 'supply chain', and not as isolated islands of efficiency.
- This applies all the more to connections between the NHS and social services in, for example, the care of the elderly.
- Success should be judged on a balance of criteria, not just on financial or budgeting success.

- Relational relationships, not control-based relationships, are the foundation of significant and successful organisational practices.
- Financial measures are only one measure of success.
- The aim is for long-term relationships with customers, although customers may be increasingly sophisticated and fickle.
- Barriers separating internal departments need to be addressed.
- Relationships involve three incremental levels of trust, namely a legal or quasi-legal *contractual trust, competence trust* and generated *goodwill trust.*
- Innovation is to be welcomed – and from any source, either internal or external.
- All employees are important to the organisation and should have the power to challenge processes if they identify a potential quality issue.

References

1   Rose MB (1994) The family firm in British business, 1780–1914. In: MW Kirby and MB Rose (eds) *Business Enterprise in Modern Britain: from the eighteenth to the twentieth century.* Routledge, London.
2   Smith A (1776) *The Wealth of Nations. Volume 1.* Methuen, London.
3   Taylor FW (1917) *The Principles of Scientific Management.* Harper and Brothers, New York.
4   Galbraith JK (1977) *The Age of Uncertainty.* BBC Worldwide Ltd, London.
5   Young JT (1997) *Economics as a Moral Science: the political economy of Adam Smith.* Edward Elgar, Cheltenham.
6   Checkland SG (1979) *The Rise of Industrial Society in England, 1815–1885.* Longman, Harlow.
7   Womack JP, Jones DT and Roos D (1990) *The Machine that Changed the World.* Rawson Associates, New York.
8   Slack N, Chambers S, Harland C, Harrison A and Johnston R (1995) *Operations Management.* Pitman Publishing, London.
9   Womack JP and Jones DT (1996) *Lean Thinking: banish waste and create wealth in your corporation.* Simon and Schuster, New York.
10 Fukuyama F (1996) *Trust: the social virtues and the creation of prosperity.* Penguin, Harmondsworth.
11 Piercy N (1997) *Market-Led Strategic Change: transforming the process of going to market* (2e). Butterworth-Heinemann, Oxford.
12 Payne A (2000) Relationship marketing: managing multiple markets. In: Cranfield School of Management (eds) *Marketing Management: a relationship marketing perspective.* Macmillan Business, London.
13 Kay N (2000) The growth of firms. In: N Foss and V Mahnke (eds) *Competence, Governance and Entrepreneurship: advances in economic strategy research.* Oxford University Press, Oxford.
14 Hines P, Lamming R, Jones D, Cousins P and Rich N (2000) *Value Stream Management: strategy and excellence in the supply chain.* Financial Times and Prentice Hall, London.

15 Sako M (1992) *Prices, Quality and Trust: inter-firm relations in Britain and Japan.* Cambridge University Press, Cambridge.

16 Kaplan RS and Norton DP (1996) *The Balanced Scorecard: translating strategy into action.* Harvard Business School Press, Boston, MA.

PART 3

The future

The liberty, prosperity and equality that are characteristic of modern capitalist societies depend crucially on maintaining a balance between self-interest and social cohesion. Historically, this balance appears to have been achieved most especially through the legal entity of the Trust. Many of our most significant social institutions have in fact been constituted as Trusts. Trusts have often acted as uniquely valuable repositories of social capital in a way that other legal entities have not. The question remains as to how contemporary healthcare trusts can engender the fellowship, loyalty and affection which have hitherto been associated with the Trust form of organisation.

Today's culture is suspicious of authority. In this context, finding new ways of establishing trust is a complex task. So we return to Piotr Sztompka's model of trust to offer ways of rebuilding primary trust, secondary trust, the trusting impulse and a trust culture. Our current situation is one of 'enlightened suspicion'. We cannot return to older attitudes of deference to professionals and 'blind trust' in authority figures. Rather, what we propose are various means of fostering an attitude of 'enlightened trust'.

Health is a 'service' in which both practitioner and patient work together to achieve an outcome. Health is not a 'product' about which we appropriately expect a measure of 'confidence'. We are concerned with an encounter of whole persons in a healing relationship where mutual trust is of the essence. 'Enlightened trust' will be characterised by shared decision making, co-production, mutuality and a virtue which may be termed 'constancy'.

Rebuilding trust will require creative thinking and action at the level of individual professionals (doctors, nurses, managers), the healthcare system (practice, primary care trust, hospital) and the institution of the NHS as a whole. The apparatus of increased accountability, by contrast, often serves mainly to increase suspicion. Rebuilding trust is an urgent and serious task in which professional groups in particular will have to take a lead.

CHAPTER 15

Macfarlane on trust and Trusts

Rob Innes

It was the Trust – and the trust which it engendered – which provided
the foundation for modern liberty, wealth and equality.

(FW Maitland)

This chapter outlines the contention of Professor Alan Macfarlane that the
'Trust' form of organisation, and the trust that it engendered, have been of
pivotal importance for the emergence of modern societies, and it examines
the continuing significance of trust and Trusts in contemporary healthcare.

Alan Macfarlane is Professor of Anthropological Science at Cambridge University.
Much of his recent writing has been concerned with the emergence of capitalism,
and the conditions needed for the emergence of contemporary liberal, capitalist
societies across the world. In *The Riddle of the Modern World*,[1] he tries to find
answers to this question with reference to four great thinkers, namely Montesquieu, Adam Smith, De Tocqueville and Ernest Gellner. In his most recent book, *The
Making of the Modern World: visions from the west and from the east*,[2] Macfarlane
focuses on one figure from the western world – the great nineteenth-century legal
historian FW Maitland. Macfarlane's study of Maitland is much more than it might
at first seem. He wishes to present Maitland not merely as a legal historian, but as a
political theorist or even a comparative sociologist – and one whose sociology
subverts much of the currently established sociological wisdom concerning the rise
of contemporary civilisation. Thus Macfarlane offers us a persuasive account of the
modern world as told by Montesquieu, Smith, De Tocqueville and Maitland, and
against the received sociological wisdom of Tönnies, Durkheim and Marx. Central
to the telling of the story is the place of 'trust' and 'Trusts'.

Macfarlane suggests that modern capitalist societies depend on maintaining a
tension between competition and co-operation – between what Adam Smith
called 'self-love and social'. A state of free competition is insufficient. This only
leads to Hobbes' 'nasty, brutish and short' life. On the other hand, the complete
fusing of everyone into one unified whole is not satisfactory either – leading in
extreme cases to the likes of Hitler, Stalin, Mao or Pol Pot. Many sociologists
(following Tönnies) have supposed that the development of modern society
involves a step change from a primitive society based on emotion, status, blood
ties and place (*Gemeinschaft* or community) to a developed society based on
contract and reason (*Gesellschaft* or partnership). However, Macfarlane argues that

modern society needs *both*. It has to find a way of fusing the two opposing human drives, and the two types of human association. This is, he suggests, precisely what 'fellowship' or 'trust' does.

The achievement of Macfarlane's most recent work is to present – through his own detailed research into the history of one English parish, and more especially through his research on Maitland – a historical account of how this actually happened. He argues rather convincingly that (in England at least) there in fact was no step change from 'peasant' civilisation to capitalist civilisation, from 'status' to 'contract', or from village community to industrial society. There was instead a gradual evolution of patterns of association from AD 1200 onwards. These developments were sustained through the evolution of English common law. Similar developments were not seen on the continent at least in part because of the widespread imposition of Roman law there.

Maitland, the great legal historian, argued that English law allowed (in a way that continental law typically did not) for the emergence of intermediary institutions between the individual and the State. Pre-eminent among these was the Trust. In the Trust form of organisation a group of individuals are able both to fulfil their own ambitions and to work co-operatively for some greater cause. The Trust offers a middle way between pure individualism and relationships based on *contract*. It offers a flexible form of association between the family business and the State-sponsored corporation. It is, in Maitland's view, a very peculiar and remarkable entity. Moreover, because it seems to bridge the gap between people and things, it could not, he believed, have arisen in countries governed under Roman law, since Roman law distinguishes sharply between people and things.

> The idea of a Trust is so familiar to us all that we never wonder at it. And yet surely we ought to wonder. If we were asked what is the greatest and most distinctive achievement performed by Englishmen in the field of jurisprudence, I cannot think that we should have any better answer to give than this, namely, the development from century to century of the Trust system.[3]

In fact, the Trust form of organisation supported the rise of many pivotal English institutions from the sixteenth century onwards (e.g. building societies, non-conformist churches, universities, the Inns of Court, numerous guilds and charities, the stock exchange, operatic societies). The Trust is an embodied entity larger than the individual, recruiting on choice or merit (not status), tolerated by the institutions of State, religion and family, and providing a sense of mutual sharing and co-operation in pursuit of some good. Trusts are, suggests Macfarlane, 'like middle-sized plants, filling in densely the space between the high vegetation, the tree-tops of State and Church, and the single individuals or family on the forest floor. ... Democracy, liberty, equality and wealth all have their roots in this common bed of associations.'[4]

If Macfarlane's theory is correct, it has several important consequences for the organisation of healthcare. First, 'trust' is not a dispensable commodity which modern society can be expected to outgrow as it becomes increasingly dependent on 'contracts'. On the contrary, capitalist society, for its own flourishing, depends crucially on the notion of trust for harmonising individual gain with social co-operation. This has many implications, but at least it undermines any supposition that the NHS would be a 'better' organisation if it downplayed the softer quality of trust in favour of the harder reality of target-related contracts.

Secondly, the Trust form of organisation ought to be celebrated over and above other forms of association such as the public limited company or the Department of State. The Trust has the rather unique ability to fuse the human qualities of warmth and solidarity with the pursuit of personal gain. Trusts act as repositories of 'social capital' in a way that other forms of organisation do not. The NHS has become one of our central social institutions, and it is an institution in which warmth and goodwill could be expected to be especially well related to its 'product', namely the healing of patients. Therefore the Trust might be expected to be a particularly apt form of organisation for the delivery of healthcare, with qualities that would not be expected, for example, in a profit-making public limited company.

Thirdly, the historical form of the Trust is far more than an instrument of management and control. It is – or could be – an embodiment of trust. One of the questions posed to Government must be how it is that the new healthcare 'Trusts' mainly lack the human qualities that the Trust form of organisation traditionally safeguarded. It may well be, as Macfarlane suggests, that the building of an effective Trust is an 'art' – that is, it requires more than the application of management science. A good Trust evokes the passionate adherence of its members. How is it that the NHS used to evoke such adherence, but does so increasingly less? And what would be needed for the culture of the new Trusts to rekindle the sympathy, devotion and sense of vocation that their employees and trustees once knew and enjoyed?

- The liberty, prosperity and equality that are characteristic of modern societies depend on maintaining a balance between self-interest and social cohesion.
- Historically, this balance appears to have been achieved most especially through the British legal institution of the Trust.
- Many of our most significant social institutions have in fact been constituted as Trusts.
- Trusts act as a repository of social capital in a way that other institutions do not.
- The question remains as to how contemporary healthcare trusts can engender the fellowship, loyalty and affection which have hitherto been associated with the Trust form of organisation.

References

1 Macfarlane A (2000, 2002) *The Riddle of the Modern World.* Palgrave, Basingstoke.
2 Macfarlane A (2002) *The Making of the Modern World: visions from the west and from the east.* Palgrave, Basingstoke.
3 Maitland FW, quoted in Macfarlane A (2002), op. cit., p. 88.
4 Macfarlane A (2002), op.cit., p. 263f.

CHAPTER 16

Rebuilding trust

Jamie Harrison and Rob Innes

How can we increase trust? By being more trustworthy.

(Timothy Jenkins)

> This chapter seeks to draw together previous strands of the book, reflecting on a shift from historic *blind trust*, via today's *enlightened suspicion*, towards a refashioned *enlightened trust*.

Introduction

Trust, or its absence, has been the central theme of earlier chapters of this book. Arguments persist over whether trust in healthcare professionals, especially doctors, has significantly decreased. Individuals continue to consult in the surgery, undergo operations and take medications.[1] Yet the public at large (in dialogue with the media) appears to be uneasy about the performance of the health service as a whole.

This chapter seeks to explore the theme of rebuilding trust. This may, of course, be the task of each and every generation, for surely there have always been scandals and public debacles. Yet today's culture is different. So we must look for contemporary ways of maintaining and, if possible, increasing public and personal trust in healthcare and its professionals. Philosophers,[2,3] sociologists[4,5] and social anthropologists[6,7] all have a part to play in the discussion. In addition, we have drawn on the experience of two recent conferences which addressed particular aspects of the debate, namely *Should We Trust Our Doctors?*,[8] and *Beyond Bristol: improving health care*,[9] which both took place in London in the autumn of 2002.

The cultural setting

In Chapter 2, on the nature of trust, Rob Innes refers to the idea that we have moved from 'a society based on fate to one based on risk'. Thus, rather than living in a universe based on providence (blind trust), we have moved to one based on risk and its estimation (enlightened suspicion). We now 'place a bet' on possible outcomes, and so make our choices. Being more calculating, and hence suspicious, we remain cautious. Being unable to work out and weigh all risks accurately, we are inevitably disappointed when things go wrong, and we may look for someone to blame.

This approach sounds very contemporary. Yet as long ago as 1784, Emmanuel Kant was encouraging people to 'Dare to use your own understanding'.[10] For Kant, no generation ought to be bound by the creeds and dogmas of past generations, but should emerge from such self-inflicted immaturity. Although his main focus was religion, it is not difficult to transfer such thinking to other external authorities. Colin Brown makes the following comment:

> His scepticism cast a long shadow over the nineteenth century. Kant personifies modern man's confidence in the power of reason to grapple with material things *and its incompetence to deal with anything beyond* (my italics).[11]

It has taken many decades for the Enlightenment critique of authority to work itself out in popular culture. Yet in our day the effects are all around us. We no longer bring up our children to defer to authority figures simply by virtue of their position. We teach our children to question and to expect rational justification for the answers that they are given. A healthy level of scepticism (or suspicion) is regarded as a good thing. And this has profound implications for the kind of trust we might seek to establish between practitioners and patients.

Some sociologists have spoken of a transition from a 'status-based' to a 'contract-based' society (such as John Newton in Chapter 10 of this book). Others have argued against this kind of step-jump in patterns of social relating (*see* Chapter 15). In the business world, we may actually be seeing a degree of disenchantment with contracts, and a search for new modes of trusting relationship (*see* Chapter 14). Whatever we make of this picture, it is evident that relationships between people who hold different levels of power and position are now much more complicated than they used to be. And in a culture of suspicion, finding new ways of establishing trust is proving to be a complex task.

Sztompka's model of trust

In his magisterial study, Piotr Sztompka constructs a powerful and wide-ranging sociological model of trust (*see* Chapter 2). For Sztompka, trust has four principal components, namely primary trust and secondary trust (associated with the trusted person), cultural trust (derived from the social environment) and the trusting impulse (a property of the one who is placing trust). We shall now consider healthcare (and some of the insights offered in previous chapters of this book) in the light of Sztompka's model.

Primary trust

Timothy Jenkins' comment that trustworthiness leads to increased trust is both self-evident and challenging. For too long, practitioners have relied on their own status. This position is no longer sustainable. People today question those in authority and take a view on such issues as reputation, performance and appearance.

- *Reputation* (*see* Chapter 10) is determined by the interplay of personal, professional and institutional standing. Reputation is a vital means for individuals to manage the risk that they bear in seeking advice from a professional person. The standing of the medical profession remains high, but patients ask themselves questions. What have they heard about this particular doctor, nurse, practice or hospital? What was their neighbour's experience? How easy is it to get an appointment and, more importantly, will they be listened to? Will their problem be taken seriously and appropriate action taken? How has it been for them in the past?

- With regard to *performance*, of course patients expect technical competence, but is there real communication, understanding and integrity in the consultation (*see* Chapter 1)? Is information being shared with them carefully and appropriately (*see* Chapter 12)? To what degree is the patient's autonomy respected? Does it feel as if they are a respected participant in the discussion?
- The *appearance* of hospital and surgery buildings (*see* Chapter 13) in terms of cleanliness and environment may promote or undermine trust. Yet healthcare is embodied more especially by its practitioners. Does what they say, in terms of words and by way of body language, encourage trust?

Secondary trust

Trust also depends on the context in which people and institutions operate. Sztompka offers three main conditions of secondary trust, namely accountability, pre-commitment and situation.

- *Accountability* can encourage trust by means of monitoring and openness. I may be more likely to trust in circumstances where practitioners know it is in their interest to prove that they are trustworthy. Yet 'hyper-accountability', as much accountability is experienced in the health service (*see* Chapter 6), may be counter-productive, and for all concerned:

  > The new accountability is ... distorting the proper aims of profes-
  > sional practice and indeed damaging professional pride and integrity.
  > Much professional practice used to centre on interaction with those
  > whom professionals serve: patients and pupils, students, and families
  > in need. Now there is less time to do this because everyone has to
  > record the details of what they do.[1]

  In addition, patients may fear, for example, that their doctor's accountability for staying within budget leads to rationing, and thus to their not receiving a particular (expensive) treatment. Adopting 'clever' accountability would cut through a bean-counting mentality (i.e. what can easily be counted) to address the real issues that worry people (i.e. what should be counted and how).
- *Pre-commitment* is the concept of a willingness to agree to actions beyond what is normally expected. If this becomes a contractual matter, such an agreement can actually reduce trust. After all, if it is set in stone, then why should I bother to trust? For trust is about mutuality, integrity and vulnerability, rather than about contract, mechanistic relationships and legalism. Where, for instance, doctors and patients sit down together to enter into a form of covenant, consenting to a mutual commitment to honesty, openness and working together,[12] then this indeed is an additional demonstration of trust. This might also be about a willingness to be together until the patient's death – the *amicus mortis* of old.[13]

- *Situation* refers to the social context. Sztompka notes that it is easier to trust in small close-knit intimate communities than in anonymous urban crowds. In addition, members of local communities are 'visible' to one another, and therefore breaches of trust are more obvious. There is evidence that patients appreciate small local practices rather than larger units (although it should be noted that in the case of Harold Shipman's single-handed practice, such trust was severely misplaced).

The trusting impulse

Psychological factors predispose some people to be more trusting than others. Early experiences in the home, within the wider family and at school shape the 'trusting impulse' – that is, the tendency people have to trust both other people and institutions. The formation of such a tendency depends on a range of factors, including a supportive family and home life, schools which model trusting relationships, and an environment in which public discourse on matters of ethics, morality and belief can flourish.

Glyn Elwyn, at the *Beyond Bristol* conference[9] referred to earlier, made a plea for practitioners to communicate at a deeper level with their patients, finding ways to explain risk and share decision making, particularly where there were major issues of uncertainty. His encouragement to 'Dare to inform', allied to Kant's 'Dare to understand', opens up the possibility of meaningful discourse right across the spectrum of health and disease, of treatments and their risks. Such an environment should provoke trust that is based on mutual acceptance and patience.

This is the kind of commitment that Alasdair Macintyre identifies in the writings of Jane Austen as 'constancy'. Commitment and responsibilities to the future spring from past episodes where obligations were conceived and debts assumed, and unite present to past to future as a unity. Macintyre notes that:

> By the time Jane Austen writes, that unity can no longer be treated as a mere presupposition or context for a virtuous life. It has itself to be continually reaffirmed, and its reaffirmation in deed rather than word is the virtue Jane Austen calls constancy.[3]

Emerging varieties of trust may be met or breached, rewarded or violated. Where trust is consistently affirmed, the trusting impulse slowly roots itself in the personality. Where it is repeatedly breached, the trusting impulse may never shape itself, or it may become suppressed, intimidated or paralysed. 'Constancy' denotes that quality of steadfastness and fidelity in a relationship which makes it feel safe to trust.

Trust culture

Trust culture is the product of institutional and national history, and is about collective memory. It affects relationships in different ways and at different levels. The patient may trust the practitioner but not the hospital or the wider health service. Those working within the NHS may not trust their managers, and vice versa. Organisations dealing with healthcare, such as social services, may be suspicious. And many may be cautious about the Government, which in turn worries about the professions. Trust breeds trust, and a culture of trust becomes self-enhancing. Equally, systematic distrust reinforces itself rapidly – once distrust has set in, it soon becomes impossible to know whether trust was ever in fact justified. The key is to engender consistent and repeated manifestations of trust so that a virtuous cycle of ever-increasing systems of trust prevails.

In Chapter 14, Robin McKenzie explored two models of business organisation – the first 'traditional' one exhibiting top-down control, and the second 'contemporary' one based on relational trust. He showed how a business culture based on trust permeates all aspects of an enterprise's dealings with its customers and suppliers, its internal production processes and, most importantly, its capacity to innovate. McKenzie argued that 'relational' businesses tend to perform significantly better than 'control-based' businesses, and he offered some pointers for what this might mean in terms of the culture of healthcare provision.

In Chapter 11, Jenny Firth-Cozens spoke of a health service culture which is too often experienced as one of 'blame, shame and punishment'. She pleaded for a culture in which people feel able to report errors, and in which there may be genuine learning from mistakes. She argued that cultural change requires leadership that has ability, benevolence and integrity.

Such change is extremely difficult, given the sensitivity of the issues involved and the wider public climate that often encourages scapegoating and litigation. However, it must be attempted if the process of learning from errors is to be sustained and the mistakes of the past avoided in the future. At the *Beyond Bristol* conference, Sir Ian Kennedy argued that 'cultural change is crucial',[9] both for the structures of healthcare and for the professionals concerned, 'allowing those who dedicate their lives to look after others the ability to do that'. He set out four propositions, namely a move from tribalism to teamwork, from blame and defensiveness to openness and accountability, from ignorance to information, and from division to understanding between clinicians and management (*see* Box 16.1). His plea recognises the need for leadership, which can redefine relationships within the health service and inspire a culture of trust.

Box 16.1   Four propositions for cultural change

- From tribalism to teamwork
- From blame and defensiveness to openness and accountability
- From ignorance to information
- From division to understanding between clinicians and management

Source: Sir Ian Kennedy[9]

The way ahead: from enlightened suspicion to enlightened trust

One key theme of the conference entitled *Should We Trust Our Doctors?*[8] was that of the need for confidence, particularly the confidence of patients in the treatment that they would receive. Among some there was also a desire to abandon talk of 'trust' in favour of the language of 'confidence'.

However, the idea of 'confidence' is itself disputed. Some sociologists take it to be a measure of reliable expectation of the delivery of a product. Others consider confidence to be an emotion of general assurance, to be contrasted with doubt.[4] What we are arguing for here is the importance of holding on to the much fuller notion of 'trust'. We are reluctant to allow that health can be reduced to the level of a commodity, such that one could be 'confident' of the product in the way that an aircraft-engine manufacturer might be confident of the dimensions and tolerance of each and every ball-bearing delivered by his supplier.

Production or co-production?

There is a critical distinction to be made here between 'goods' and 'services'. Goods are tangible economic products that are capable of being touched, tasted and consumed. Services are more akin to 'acts' – of kindness, advice or support – where there is 'consumer/client' involvement before, during and after the offering of the service. The characteristics of services include intangibility, inseparability and variability (*see* Box 16.2).

Box 16.2   Features of a service industry

- *Intangibility*. Clients may have little evidence in advance of what to expect, limited understanding of the complex processes involved, and be unclear what has actually happened (e.g. car servicing, buying a pension, consulting a doctor).
- *Inseparability*. Services are produced with customers (co-production) rather than separately in a factor (*see also* Box 16.3).
- *Variability*. An inevitable consequence of simultaneous production and consumption is the variability in performance of the service (unlike the production line).

Source: Urban Partnership Group. London School of Economics and Political Science (2001); http://www.wholesystems.co.uk

---

While wishing to resist notions of 'health' as a commodity, the idea of co-production may be helpful as a way of explaining interactions in service relationships, particularly in contradistinction to models of industrial production. The notion of 'co-production' highlights the experience of being served – the customer/client is present at the point of production (unlike the purchaser of a motor car), participates with the producer in consumption of the service, and will revisit that experience at a later date (*see* Box 16.3).

This model of co-production can be expressed in diagrammatic form (*see* Box 16.4), where the engagement of the clinician with the patient is represented in the central column of the box. Different patients will wish to engage with

---

Box 16.3 Features of co-production

- Relationalism
- Imparting expertise/information
- Co-operation
- Balance of control
- Balance of authority
- Flexibility of approach

Source: Notes from a seminar by Richard Normann, Urban Partnership Group, London School of Economics and Political Science (2001).

---

different levels of co-production, depending on their own knowledge, personality and experiences. Equally, a patient who is very unwell may wish the doctor to 'take control', whereas on other occasions that same patient would wish to be an equal partner in decision making (*see* Box 16.4 and also van Zwanenberg[14]).

Box 16.4 Decision making in the consultation with patients

Professional choice	*Shared decision making*	*Consumer choice*
Clinician decides	Information shared	Clinician informs
	Values clarified	
Patient consents	Joint decision	Patient decides

Source: Angela Coulter[9] and http://www.pickereurope.org

Engaging with the whole person

At the end of Chapter 1, Ruth Etchells made a plea for a return to the 'human dimension'. She reflected on the implications of that for her, which included opening a dialogue with the Government over doctor numbers, establishing a culture of admitting mistakes, patients becoming aware of what is realistically possible, and recognising the doctor as a human being with personal needs.

Traditional professional training has encouraged practitioners of all types to see patients as a whole. The above agenda also challenges patients to reflect on their own portion of the 'bargain', and to engage in encounters beyond what might be seen as their own limited self-interest. In such relationships, the risks of mutual openness, vulnerability and possible failure abound. Yet to exclude such risks may render these interactions mechanical, uninspired and potentially sterile.

> Doctors and nurses in healthcare settings exercise professional judgement using their skills and training, but they are whole personalities, and quality, as perceived by their clients, is determined by their whole approach. Holism is a two-way street in which the whole clinician deals with the whole patient.[15]

Normann goes on to comment that, all too often, ideas such as 'bedside manner' are interpreted as being marginal compared with 'real' quality as defined by therapeutic efficiency and clinical outcome. This is a mistake, particularly when the transactions relate to the provision of 'care' in which enhancement of well-being is the primary objective. How the patient feels ('the subjective perceptions of the interaction held by the customer') is then a critical measure of the quality of such transactions.

The concept of enlightened trust

The days of blind trust are surely over. Yet the current experience of enlightened suspicion, with its hyper-accountability, inspection visits, targets, quality measures, performance indicators, league-tables and systems of inspection (with threats of punitive interventions) demotivates and paralyses professionals, and diminishes trust.

> Punitive inspection does not produce a climate that fosters trust, learning and improved performance. And as it is based on a model of mistrust and suspicion, it is unlikely to achieve the desired results.[16]

Calls for transparency and accountability need careful qualification. What does 'transparency' mean? And how is information to be properly interpreted and balanced in a very complex system?[2] Accountability is essential, but how is it to be made 'clever' – that is, meaningful, sensible and appropriate to the task? Equally, although patients need to feel confidence in their practitioners and health service, that is only a part of the story. Building confidence bilaterally leads to enduring trusting relationships – a more developed and beneficial state for all concerned.

Building enlightened trust

Ultimately trust must be earned. Demonstrating trustworthiness, constancy and openness is a beginning, yet these need the support of good systems, effective teams and appropriate leadership. There also needs to be a cultural change, both for individuals and for their organisations (*see* Box 16.5).

Box 16.5   From blind trust to enlightened suspicion to enlightened trust

Blind trust	*Enlightened suspicion*	*Enlightened trust*
Acceptance	Questioning	Shared decisions
Receptivity	Consumption	Co-production
Passivity	Accountability	Mutuality
Ignorance	Inspection	Information
Dependence	Confidence	Constancy

Trust in the individual (doctor, nurse or manager)

Recall our opening quotation: 'How can we increase trust? By being more trustworthy.' Individual practitioners are shaped by their training (*see* Chapter 9), peer group and life experiences. Ethical codes and their modern equivalents may have a place in setting out the standards of trustworthy behaviour, but the more fundamental issue is the formation of individuals who are trustworthy. Right action proceeds from right desires and right character attributes.

Much recent ethical thinking in medicine is rooted either in *deontology* (using notions of obligations and duties, e.g. the General Medical Council's *Duties of a Doctor*[17]) or in *utilitarianism* (weighing costs and benefits, e.g. the drive towards evidence-based practice). However, the philosophical renaissance of *virtue ethics* (associated in particular with Alasdair Macintyre, but going back originally to Aristotle and Plato) surely has a significant place in the discussion. Indeed, this case has recently been argued by Peter Toon.[18]

Toon wants to encourage a rather fundamental examination of what it means to be 'a good doctor'. In the tradition of virtue ethics, this would mean the person leading a good and fulfilling life, both at work and outside work. It would involve cultivating the central Aristotelian virtue of 'Practical Wisdom', and using this to judge other desirable virtues such as courage, temperance, benevolence and justice. It would involve the pursuit of moral and rational excellence, and it would also entail reflection on the qualities to be encouraged in 'a good patient'.

In this light, Toon sees the essence of the doctor–patient relationship not so much as 'rational beneficence' but as a holistic encounter of thinking and feeling persons:

> To do what is right for patients is not a matter of respecting their autonomy and acting beneficently towards them, but involves trying to see things from their perspective, understand what they are feeling with our feelings, and not just doing good to them but liking them (especially when they are particularly dislikeable).[18]

Perhaps many doctors and patients would like consultations to have this empathetic quality, while recognising that current practice is often much more functional in nature. Renewing the teaching of ethics (*see* Chapter 9) and exploring the experience of human relationships through literature and the arts[19] (*see* Chapter 7), both within training programmes and beyond, offers one way of beginning to address these fundamental issues.

Trust in the system (practice, primary care trust or hospital)

John Donne tells us that no individual is 'an island'. All who work in the health service do so as part of a wider grouping (clinical team, management unit or professional body), yet isolation and marginalisation remain constant risks for team members. Creating and sustaining teams according to the model of the 'relational' companies identified in Chapter 14 offers one way forward. Yet the target-driven control culture of the NHS compromises such a move. Managers in particular fear for their jobs should they fail to deliver on the latest initiative from above.

> Without trust there can be no sensible way of running a complex system like the NHS. But modern trust does not entail a retreat into outmoded models of professional paternalism. Rather, it is underpinned by the values of open debate, scepticism, inquisitiveness, and the pursuit of continuous learning and improvement. All of these are in short supply when the policy context is dominated by a centralising government intent on controlling the agenda.[16]

Local organisations therefore struggle, with clinicians and managers exposed to the whims of central planners. Only by regaining some degree of local autonomy and a local mandate is movement possible. Here the primary care trusts as they were originally conceived – as local partnerships between healthcare and the public – need to gain confidence. Macfarlane[6] reminds us of the nature of the historical Trust, where mutual co-operation and sharing are central. Increasing trust and social capital, as opposed to a pure profit motivation, are crucial to the success of the Trust. For 'profit' we might suggest 'target'. In Chapter 15, Rob Innes made the telling point that although the NHS once evoked passionate adherence from its workers, now it does not do so.

Trust in the institution (the NHS)

Any discussion about healthcare in the UK will end up talking about the NHS, and any discussion about the NHS will lead to the issue of Government control (*see* Chapter 6). For the politicisation of the NHS has profound implications – for policy, culture and the workforce, and not least for patients. There is a theory that the most politicised health services around the world fare the worst.[20] Now, of course, governments have a legitimate role to play, especially in a State-funded health system, in the triumvirate of Government, healthcare system and the public. Each player contributes to and receives from the debate (an effective service, money and status, access to healthcare, and so on). Yet the power relationships may be unbalanced, not least where a government seeks to impose a style of policy, regulation and management which is destructive of trust. Equally, the professions themselves may appear untrustworthy and self-seeking, and patients may be perceived as too demanding and unrealistic. Brian Salter expresses his concerns as follows:

> If the triangular relationship between medicine, society and the State is to survive as a central component of the modern welfare state – and at present there is no alternative to this arrangement – then the decline in public trust in the profession has to be halted. ... The public has not been reassured and a common discourse has yet to be established.[21]

Although we may argue over the degree of lost trust, Salter is persuasive in his plea for a common discourse. He makes plain the dilemma of governments in their symbiotic relationships with the medical profession – either reduce the public's faith in doctors by over-aggressive posturing (and risk their inability to deliver State policy), or regulate the profession even more directly (and risk directing the wrath of the public over falling standards at themselves). He goes on to point out that citizens want to open up this closed relationship between Government and medicine, to be involved in all stages of the discussions, and to share the power equitably. However, there are doubts as to whether the State and professions are ready for this yet.[22] He ends with a note of warning:

> A more probable outcome in the short term is an attempted accommodation that merely genuflects to citizen participation, but does not confront the underlying issue. Such an outcome is unlikely to be sustainable.

In his 2002 Dimbleby Lecture, the Archbishop of Canterbury suggested that the 'nation state' is giving way to the 'market state'. The State is increasingly less able to deliver in terms of the traditional expectations of guaranteeing the general good of the community. Instead, the State's role is to 'clear a space' for groups and individuals to secure their own best deal.

> It means the Government is free to encourage enterprise not to protect against risk; to try to increase the literal and metaphorical purchasing power of its citizens but not to take for granted anything much in the way of agreement about common goods or social goods.[23]

If Rowan Williams is right, then this makes the delivery of real government leadership with respect to the NHS problematic. For the NHS has traditionally been the flagship of an agreed 'common good' within the post-World War Two Welfare State. Williams' point is that governments increasingly struggle to articulate the values which underpin such goods in a way that commands active assent from their electorates.

The trend towards a 'market state' does not necessarily mean that the NHS would be inevitably destined eventually to be replaced by a 'market' in healthcare. However, it does mean, surely, that professional and producer groups will have to provide a stronger and fuller rationale and ethos for the health service, and be able to articulate this in the public arena. Professional leadership may need to take up what Government leadership finds it increasingly difficult to deliver.

Crucially, this will mean professional groups developing strong and productive relationships with the local and national press. Very frequently the press have been seen as 'the bad guys'. In Chapter 8, Louella Houldcroft reminded us that the press is itself bound by strict ethical codes. Professional groups need to work with journalists both to promote individual success and to expose problems with the NHS that affect us all. By proactively feeding information to the press, a hospital or health centre can raise its profile as well as boosting the confidence of the patients who use it. Even when bad news is reported, the press fulfils an important function in protecting the public interest and in forcing debate and action from those responsible.

Conclusion

Rebuilding trust will not mean 'more of the same'. All has changed, and each of the parties in the relationship must move on. Doctors can no longer assume that they are trusted. They must demonstrate trustworthiness, and over time. Patients also need assurance that they are seen as whole people, engaging in real discourses – not just by the health system but also by the State. Governments must heed the warnings of O'Neill and others that their drive for so-called transparency, account-ability and micro-management is ultimately futile and destructive of trust.

The concept of trust, with its connotations of mutuality, confidence, vulnerability and reasonable hope, is one to be valued and not disparaged. If there truly is a 'crisis of trust',[2] then rebuilding trust should be an urgent and serious endeavour for all.

- A culture of increasing suspicion has replaced blind trust.
- Therefore trust can no longer be assumed, but must be earned.
- Responses to suspicion include hyper-accountability and micro-management, both of which further undermine trust.
- A new, enlightened trust accepts the need for openness and reason, but demands mutuality and vulnerability in relationships.
- Ultimately, it is only by being trustworthy that people can be trusted.

References

1   O'Neill O (2002) *Is Trust Falling? Reith Lecture 2;* http://www.bbc.co.uk/radio4/reith2002
2   O'Neill O (2002) *A Question of Trust. The BBC Reith Lectures 2002.* Cambridge University Press, Cambridge.
3   Macintyre A (1985) *After Virtue: a study in moral theory.* Duckworth, London.
4   Sztompka P (1999) *Trust. A sociological theory.* Cambridge University Press, Cambridge.
5   Beck U, Giddens A and Lash S (1994) *Reflexive Modernization.* Polity Press, Cambridge.
6   Macfarlane A (2002) *The Making of the Modern World: visions from the west and from the east.* Palgrave, Basingstoke.
7   Jenkins T (1999) *Religion in English Everyday Life.* Berghahn Books, New York.
8   Royal Society of Medicine (2002) *Should We Trust Our Doctors?* Conference held on 30 and 31 October, London.
9   *Beyond Bristol: improving health care.* British Medical Association Conference held on 18 November 2002, London.
10   Kant E (1784) *What is Enlightenment?* Berlinische Monatsschrift, Berlin.
11   Brown C (1969) *Philosophy and the Christian Faith. A historical sketch from the middle ages to the present day.* Inter-Varsity Press, London.
12   Harrison J (2001) The world in which we live. In: J Harrison, R Innes and T van Zwanenberg (eds) *The New GP.* Radcliffe Medical Press, Oxford.
13   Illich I (1995) Death undefeated. *BMJ.* **311**: 1652–3.
14   van Zwanenberg T (2001) The new GP. In: J Harrison, R Innes and T van Zwanenberg (eds) *The New GP.* Radcliffe Medical Press, Oxford.
15   Urban Partnership Group (2001) *Service Industries, Health Care and Systems Reconfiguration.* Notes from a seminar given by Richard Normann, London

School of Economics and Political Science, London. See also Normann R (1991) *Service Management.* John Wiley & Sons, New York.

16   Calman K, Hunter DJ and May A (2002) *Make or Break Time? A commentary on Labour's health policy two years into the NHS Plan.* University of Durham School for Health, Stockton on Tees.

17   General Medical Council (2001) *Duties of a Doctor.* General Medical Council, London.

18   Toon P (2002) The sovereignty of virtue. *Br J Gen Pract.* **52**: 694–5.

19   Macnaughton J (2002) Arts and humanities in medical education. In: J Harrison and T van Zwanenberg (eds) *GP Tomorrow* (2e). Radcliffe Medical Press, Oxford.

20   Smith R (2002) Oh NHS, thou art sick. The NHS's main problem may be overpoliticisation. *BMJ.* **324**: 127–8.

21   Salter B (2000) *Medical Regulation and Public Trust. An international review.* King's Fund Publishing, London.

22   Smith R (2002) The discomfort of patient power. Medical authorities will have to live with 'irrational' decisions by the public. *BMJ.* **324**: 497–8.

23   Williams R (2002) The 2002 Dimbleby Lecture. *The Times.* **19 December**.

CHAPTER 17

Conclusion

Jamie Harrison

> We have all been more or less to blame.
> (Jane Austen, *Mansfield Park*, 1814)

> The land had not changed. ... Only, the times ... they had changed.
> (Ford Madox Ford, *Parade's End*, 1928)

There are risks in harbouring yearnings for a disappearing past. In their different ways, both Jane Austen's *Mansfield Park* and Ford Madox Ford's *Parade's End* embody and explore the shift in sensibility from one century to the next. As we enter the new, twenty-first century, certainties of a previous era are under suspicion, and ways of experiencing relationships are under review. Trust – or the lack of it – has become a key issue.

In such a context, it is tempting to retreat into nostalgia and defensiveness. Blaming someone else for the failures and misunderstandings that inevitably arise in everyday discourse becomes easy. The consequent loss of trust is then difficult to repair. Wittgenstein likened rebuilding such lost trust to the job of refashioning a broken spider's web.

In this book we have argued that all players in the world of healthcare are important, whether they are patients, politicians or professionals. Each grouping has a responsibility to participate, and to do so with confidence but not arrogance. Equally, both the media and the wider public have legitimate and necessary contributions to make to the debate, not least on matters of trust. This concluding chapter will reflect briefly on possible ways ahead, moving from a culture of increasing suspicion to one of greater trust.

Questioning or shared decisions?

Who holds the power in medical decision making? For too long, patients have found themselves mere observers in their consultations with doctors, with little encouragement to ask questions, interact and share in what might take place. Although change is occurring, it can be slow and tortuous. While there may be occasions when patients prefer others to make the decisions for them, this increasingly appears to be the exception rather than the rule.

Consumption or co-production?

Is healthcare a commodity to be bought and sold? In answering this question, it is easy for professionals to become self-righteous in proclaiming the special, non-commercial nature of health, and their role in maintaining it. This avoids the need for efficiency or market sensitivity. The concept of co-production encourages thinking of 'health' as a joint effort between patient and practitioner, based on trust and co-operation.

Accountability or mutuality?

Who is accountable in the world of healthcare, and to whom? Traditional models suggest that doctors are accountable only to themselves, with the public and parliament looking on from a distance. Recent tragic events have altered this dynamic. However, mutual accountability within the triad of patient, politician and professional might offer a far better way for the future.

Inspection or information?

Is a system of inspection the right way to change behaviour and improve outcomes? Recent explorations of this theme would suggest that the opposite is the case, with all parties becoming frustrated and upset by failures to make progress. Proper mechanisms for gathering the right healthcare information could allow both proper debate and a new culture of reflection and improvement, as part of a learning organisation, to develop.

Confidence or constancy?

Where a doctor is trusted, how much depends on a belief in the doctor's professional competence and how much depends on the perception that the doctor is committed to the patient as a person? Both aspects, of course, lead to confidence in the practitioner. Yet a technically expert doctor may never have learned empathy for the patient, just as a sympathetic doctor may be incompetent. Constancy suggests a track record in commitment and mutual understanding, with an agreement to see things through. It must also mean commitment to keeping up to date.

Suspicion or trust?

Will there be increasing suspicion or greater trust? An increased willingness to question appropriately can go hand in hand with a greater desire for openness – and this applies to everyone. Trustworthy practitioners allay patients' fear. Patients also need to see their practitioners as human beings. This will be about a new dialogue – between people who are prepared to trust one another.

Edmund's confession in *Mansfield Park* in the opening quote – that the family had failed their father in his absence – is a pivotal moment in the novel, and a poignant reminder of how easily enthusiasm can turn to impropriety. All changes, and something of the innocence of *Mansfield Park* is lost for ever. There are therefore parallels with our world of medicine, where the trust between doctors and their patients has been questioned as a result of much-publicised scandals and mistakes, and where there is no going back to a previous age of naivety.

Yet Jane Austen fashions from the debacle new possibilities and new ways of being family. Trust is rebuilt through the constancy of some and the willingness of others to rethink their views and position. There is a new sensibility about, which transcends the old fixities without denying their existence.

Medicine will need to say it is sorry for past mistakes and mean it. It will also need to remember that it still retains the trust of the vast majority of the public, and that there is no better time than the present to build on that trust with confidence and integrity.

Index